MEDICO-LEGAL HANDBOOK
FOR DOCTORS

MEDICO-LEGAL HANDBOOK
FOR DOCTORS

Dr Dotun Adenugba
MBBS, MRCOG
PG. Dip Law, LLM Medical Law

Contribution by
Alison Eddy
Partner, Irwin Mitchell Solicitors

MEDICOLEGAL HANDBOOK FOR DOCTORS

Published by the legaldoc
P.O.Box 570
Herts, EN8 1EA
Email: info@thelegaldoc.co.uk

First published 2006
© Dotun Adenugba 2006

The right of Dotun Adenugba to be identified as author of this work has been asserted by her in accordance with the Copyright, Designs and Patents Act 1988.

No part of this publication may be reproduced, stored in a retrieval system, or transmitted in any form or by any means, electronic, mechanical, photocopying, recording or otherwise, without either the prior permission of the publishers or a licence permitting restricted copying in the United Kingdom issued by the Copyright Licensing Agency, 90 Tottenham Court Road, London W1T 4LP. Enquiries concerning reproduction outside the scope of the above should be sent to the publisher at the address above.

You must not circulate this book in any other binding or cover and you must impose the same condition on the subsequent purchaser.

ISBN 10: 0-9553975-0-2
ISBN 13: 978-0-9553975-0-9

British Library Cataloguing in Publication Data
A catalogue record of this book is available from the British Library

Notice
The medical law is constantly changing, with new law and developments in existing law being introduced all the time. The law is believed to be correctly stated as at May 2006. Readers are advised where necessary, to check the most current position of the law and consult a legal adviser.

This book is intended to be a general guide to medical law and not a substitute for legal advice. Neither the authors nor the publisher assumes any liability for loss to any persons or property arising from this publication.

Contents

Acknowledgement 9
Preface 10
Introduction 11
Abbreviation 13

PART 1   LEGAL RELATIONS
1. The Doctor as an Employee (who rules the rooster?) 15
2. The Doctor and the Patient (love thy neighbour!) 24

PART 2   APPLIED MEDICAL LAW & ETHICS
3. Informed Consent (the whole truth and nothing but the truth!) 54
4 Consent in Obstetrics 73
5. Confidentiality (even the walls have ears! ssssshhhhh) 81
6. End of Life Decisions (when the curtain is drawn) 106

PART 3   GOVERNANCE
7. Clinical Governance (an inspector calls!) 118
8. Clinical Risk Management (mind the gap!) 129
9. Information Governance (setting the records straight!) 137
10. Communication (look who's talking!) 143
11. Performance Management (how am I driving? Call 0800-GMC) 151

PART 4   'WHEN THINGS FALL APART'
12. Complaints - NHS & GMC Complaints Procedure 157
13. Managing complaints 162
14. Dealing with an adverse incident 167
15. Disciplinary & Grievance Procedures 170

APPENDIX

A. Synopsis of the English Legal System 175
B. Overview of a Medical Negligence Claim 184
C. Legal Case Reporting 185
D. Glossary of legal terms 187
E. NHS Structures 189
F. Duties of a Doctor Registered with the General Medical Council 196
G. The GMC guidance library 197
H. Guidance for Health Professionals on completing the Department of Health / Welsh Office Consent Form 1 198
I . Child protection guideline 202
J. Post Death Investigations (The Coroner) 204

ACKNOWLEDGEMENTS

I would like to acknowledge the contribution made to this book in the chapter on 'Consent in Obstetrics' by Alison Eddy, Partner at Irwin Mitchell Solicitors.

I would also like to thank John Bolger for his meticulous and painstaking reading of the book and the suggestions made.

To my big brother, Dr Rotimi Jaiyesimi for your time in reading through and the contributions made. I appreciate you.

Finally to all my friends and family who have supported and encouraged me to complete the book as they could not wait to get their hands on a copy ! Merci!

Preface

Where medicine and the law meet the doctor is usually at a disadvantage.

Not understanding the law as it applies to medicine can cause considerable anxiety in the doctor and affect good clinical judgements. Even in daily life the law is associated with mystique and incomprehension, its language both written and spoken impenetrable by the uninitiated. Recently however, society has entered an era where the doctor cannot be an effective clinician without a modicum of knowledge of the workings of the law.

This book is written for the doctor who feels unsure about medico-legal matters or lacks confidence when entering this area. This hand book demystifies the law. The book decodes its language and explains the concepts behind it. It shows how laws come about, how they are tested and how they are refined. With this basic knowledge the book shows how the doctor can navigate safely through the menacing waters of malpractice, research ethics, the workplace and everywhere the law has an influence.

Having read this book, the doctor will be free to treat the patient without anxiety or hampered by misconceptions

John Bolger
June 2006

INTRODUCTION

I woke up one September morning in 2004 with an intense desire to write this book. Writing a book was definitely not in the scheme of things I had planned for the year or the immediate future. The inspiration and flow of thought was overwhelming.

The impetus for this being the deep quagmire of legal pitfalls I had observed in doctors in the hospital through lack of knowledge of Medical law and Ethics.

Further, there is a paucity of basic and easy to read handbooks of medical law and ethics dealing with the poignant and ethically challenging decisions in clinical practice.

My journey to writing this book started with reviewing and reading the available books on the market. Whilst credit is given to the authors for the quality of the materials, many were complex, voluminous and did not address the quandaries of legal and ethical issues encountered in clinical practice.

The objective in writing this book is to present medical law and ethics in a readable and accessible form by setting out the general principles of the subject, addressing problem areas and contentious aspects. It is aimed at providing an inroad into the substantive and practical principles of legal and ethical issues in clinical practice.

By illustrating with caselaw, it is hoped that the reader will have a better understanding of the principles and the law .To help the reader come to grasps with the legal tone of the book, I will recommend reading the appendices A - C as a preliminary to understanding the English legal system and legal case reporting.

This handbook is intended to be a prophylactic recipe for good clinical practice, and to reduce complaints and litigation In addition, it expounds on the contractual and employment law issues for hospital doctors, the regulatory and disciplinary procedures applicable to doctors. I hope this handbook will be particularly helpful to foreign trained doctors who have got to come to grasp very quickly the ethos of the legal and ethical issues relevant to clinical practice in the U.K.

Finally no one can write any work of medical law and ethics without reference to the guidance notes / directives of the General Medical Council, the British Medical Association and the Department of Health. The contribution of these have been immense, acknowledgement is given to this fact and the help each one has given me in writing this handbook.

ABBREVIATION

Act	Act of Parliament
Art	Articles of the Human Rights Act 1998
BMA	British Medical Association
CNST	Clinical Negligence Scheme for Trusts
Dept	Department
DoH	Department of Health
EWTR	European Working Time Regulation
GMC	General Medical Council
GP	General Practitioner
HCC	HealthCare Commission
HFEA	Human Fertilisation & Embryology Authority
HSG	Health Service Guidance
NMC	Nursing & Midwifery Council
NHS	National Health Service
NHSLA	National Health Service Litigation Authority
NPSA	National Patient Safety Authority
PCT	Primary Care Trust
RCOG	Royal College of Obstetrics & Gynaecology
RCS	Royal College of Surgeons
SHO	Senior House Officer
SpR	Specialist Registrar

LEGAL RELATIONS

INTRODUCTION

The modern era of protectionism and rights has evolved to create legal relations between parties in the course of their obligations. In this chapter I intend to explore two key legal relationships of the doctor in the course of his duties:

a) with the employer and b) with his patient. In the course of the doctor's dealing with these two parties, it can be stated that there is an intention to create relations usually established by an outward indication of an agreement to do something or a subjective assessment of the actual intention of the parties.

Chapter 1
THE DOCTOR AS AN EMPLOYEE
(who rules the rooster!)

The parties to an employment relationship are the employee (a doctor) and the employer (the hospital) and arising from this relationship are legal rights and obligations under the common law and legislation. For doctors in hospital, the employer is either the NHS Trust or the Primary Care Trust if community based.

Where a doctor works as a locum through an agency, he will not be an employee but a worker. This distinction is important especially where disputes arise in relation to unfair dismissal, redundancy and maternity rights though in the dispensation of the locum doctor's duties he is under the control of the employing Trust.

The Contract of Employment

This is the document that evidences the contractual relationship between the parties. It sets out the terms and conditions of the contract, identifying the rights and duties of the parties to the contract. The main conditions of service for doctors in the NHS is set out in the Terms and Conditions of Service of Hospital Medical and Dental staff (England and Wales) (the "TCS") and the Condition of Service of the General Council of the Whitley Councils for the Health Services. These documents are notoriously long and convoluted but have been nationally agreed in the best interests of the doctors. Any contract of employment should state that it is subject to these terms and conditions. The terms cover matters such as annual leave, occupational sick pay, study leave, part time and whole time appointments. These documents form the express terms of the contract of employment by incorporation.

Further by s1 of the Employment Rights Act 1996 (ERA 1996) the contract of employment must set out within two months a written statement of the terms and conditions relating to the following matters:

- The parties to the contract
- Date and period of employment
- Job description
- Scale or rate of remuneration: There is a nationally agreed scale but doctors should ensure that the correct salary point is allocated taking into account previous years experience and service, relevant qualifications and research experience.

Band Supplements

From 1 Dec 2000, the Additional Duty Hours (ADH) pay system was replaced with a pay banding system. The bands reflect whether the post is 'New Deal' compliant, whether the doctors works up to 40, 48 or to 56 hours a week, the type of working pattern, the intensity of work and the anti-social nature of the working arrangements.

This supplement is a single sum of money, calculated as a proportion of the basic salary (see below) and added to the monthly salary to remunerate overall time on duty. There are different levels of supplement depending on the nature of the post.

This will apply to doctors and dentists including flexible trainees in the training grades. If a flexible trainee does 40hours of actual work per week or more they will be treated exactly the same as a full time trainee- allocated to a band using the same criteria as full timers and receive the full pay for that band with no pro rota reduction. Full time doctors whose entire working week consists of 40 hours or less between 8am and 7p.m, Mon-Fri, will receive no additional supplements The banding for the post should be detailed in the contract of employment

There are three bands in the new system:

a. Band 1 includes all juniors whose posts are compliant with the New Deal and who work up to and including 48hours of actual work per week.

b. Band 2 includes all juniors whose post are compliant with the New Deal and who work over 48hours and up to and including 56 hours of actual work per week.

c. Band 3 includes all juniors whose posts are non compliant with the New Deal.

Band 2 is split into Bands 2A and 2B, and Band 1 is split into Bands 1A, 1B and 1C:

i. Bands 2A and 1A includes all juniors who, within their respective hours' limits, work at a high intensity and at the most unsocial times, as defined by the banding criteria.

ii. Bands 2B and 1B includes all juniors who, within their respective hours' limit, work at less intensity and less unsocial times.

iii. Band 1C includes all juniors working on a low frequency on-call rota from home.

The total salary of junior doctors will comprise a basic salary to which a supplement, calculated as a proportion of the basic salary, will be added according to the band to which the doctor is allocated, as set out below:

Band 1A	50%	Band 2A	80%	Band FA	25%
Band 1B	40%	Band 2B	50%	Band FB	5%
Band 1C	20%	Band 3	100%	Band FC	pro-rota

An additional band F accommodates flexible trainees who work less than 40 hours of actual work per week. Band F is split into FA, FB and FC, according to the hours and pattern of work criteria. As stated above a flexible trainee who does 40 hours of actual work or more will be treated in exactly the same way as a full time trainee.

- Hours of work
- Place or places of work.
- Any terms relating to annual leave, sickness and sick pay, pension and pension schemes.
- Period of notice to terminate contract.
- Particulars of any collective agreements which directly affect the terms of employment.
- Policies e.g. disciplinary and grievance policies, sharps, equal opportunities, bullying and harassment policies.
- Whether any previous employment is taken into account as continuous employment

Any disputes about the terms of the contract or changes must be raised with the employer within a month of the change. If you do not take action quickly and continue to work under changed terms, it would be deemed that you have accepted the changes by your actions or lack of objection. It is advisable to seek advice early from the British Medical Association or a specialist employment solicitor/adviser on any disputed terms in the contract.

Implied Terms

Despite a written contract of employment, terms will be implied into a contract either at common law or under a legislation in the absence of detailed agreement. The following are examples:

By Legislation:
- The Working Time Regulations 1998
  # Weekly Hours: To work no more than 48hrs on average a week over a 17week period
  # Daily rest: A minimum of 11hours rest in between each working day.

- # Weekly rest: A minimum of 24hours each 7day week.
- # Rest breaks: A 20 minute break if you work more than 6 consecutive hours.
- Equal Pay Act 1970 inserts an equality clause to every contract of employment to ensure that women and men are remunerated equally if they do "like work".

  It is anti discriminative in its purpose. It is unlikely that differences in pay for female and male doctors will occur in NHS employment contracts.

- Health and Safety at Work Act 1974 provides the framework for modern health and safety in the workplace. It imposes a duty on the employer to ensure so far as is reasonably practicable, the health, safety and welfare at work of all his employers and on the employee to take reasonable care for the health and safety of themselves and other persons and where duties or requirements are imposed on employers, to cooperate with them to enable the duty or requirement to be carried out. All people are required not to intentionally interfere with or misuse anything which has been provided by law in the interests of health and safety (e.g fire escapes, guards or machines).

- Sick Pay Act 1994 provides that the employer must pay sick pay for the first 28days and after that the employee is entitled to state sickness benefit.

- Employment Rights Act 1996

- # Antenatal care : s55 Employment Rights Act 1996 provides the right to time off attend antenatal care to all female employees irrespective of length of service or hours of work. The employee may however be required to produce a doctor or midwife's certificate of pregnancy and appointment card

- # Paternity Leave: s80A Employment Rights Act 1996 provides for 2weeks paternity leave for each child. This must be taken before the end of the period of 56days beginning with the birth of the child. There may be conditions as to the period of employment and association with the child born.

- # Adoption Leave: Chapter 1A ERA 1996 makes provision for a new right to a period of paid adoption leave. This will apply to the adoptive parents of children placed or matched for adoption on or after 6th April 2003. The provisions mirror maternity leave below.

\# Maternity leave: Every woman is entitled to maternity leave. There are two types depending on the woman's length of service. Ordinary maternity leave is for 26weeks for all women regardless of their length of service or hours of work During this leave the woman's contract of employment continues. She is therefore entitled to the benefit of all the terms and conditions of employment except remuneration. Some women are entitled to additional maternity leave if they have a period of employment of 26weeks or more at the start of the 14th week of the pregnancy. This additional leave commences on the day after the last day of the ordinary maternity leave for up to 26weeks from the day it commenced.

By Common Law:

Terms can be implied into a contract of employment at common law. The principal implied duties are set out below under employer and employee duties.

Employer duties

- Duty to pay wages

- Duty to take reasonable care of the employee's safety and working conditions. This duty of care extends only to the employees' personal safety and not his property.

- Duty of mutual trust and confidence. The employer must cooperate with the employee and not make his task in any way more difficult. That the employer will not without reasonable cause conduct themselves in a manner calculated or likely to destroy or seriously damage the relationship of mutual trust and confidence between the employer and the employee.

The employer must not behave in a way which is intolerable or in a way which employees cannot be expected to put up with any longer. This will include failing to show respect for the employee, open rebuke and ridicule, shouting or humiliating the employee.' Woods- v- WM Car Services (Peterborough) Ltd [1983] IRLR 413, CA

- Duty to take reasonable care in giving references. The employer in compiling or giving a reference should take care to ensure the accuracy of its contents- true, accurate and fair. There is no duty to give a reference and the employee may request for copies of the reference under the Data Protection Act 1998.

- Duty to indemnify the employee for expenses and liabilities incurred by the employee in the course of his employment.

Employee Duties

The general principle is that the employee must serve the employer and his interest faithfully. The relationship of the employer and employee is a personal one and the employee may not delegate performance of his duties. The doctor must therefore exercise his or her judgement and discretion in carrying out their duties faithfully in the interest of the employer.

- Obedience to instruction: The employee is obliged to obey all lawful orders of the employer. The construction of this lawful order is entrenched in the following terms of the contract of employment:

  'It is agreed that you are liable as far as is practicable, to deputise from time to time for absent colleagues in accordance with para 108 of 'TCS''.

  "It is agreed that exceptionally you will be available for additional work in occasional emergencies and unforeseen circumstances."

  "It is agreed that exceptionally you will be available for such irregular commitments outside your normal rostered duties as are essential for the continuation of patient care."

  In the construction of these wide clauses, it is not intended to make it impossible for the doctor to have a defined set of duties. The employers' instructions must be tempered with reasonableness.

- Duty of reasonable care and indemnity : The doctor is under a duty to carry out his duties exercising reasonable care and skill. If he fails so to do, he is liable to indemnify the employer for the loss suffered by the employer by reason of the employee's breach.

- Duty of good faith: This mirrors the duty of trust and confidence by the employer. During employment the employee must not disclose confidential information. This duty is set out in the GMC guidance 'Good Medical Practice' (2001) and 'Confidentiality' : Protecting and Providing and Information.

SUMMARY

- A doctor who is employed by an employing hospital is in a contractual relationship with the hospital who is the employer.

- The parties to an employment relationship will often put the terms and conditions that govern that relationship into writing- the contract of employment

- Even where there is a written contract which sets out the express terms which govern the relationship, collective or workforce agreements (e.g. T&CS), the common law and legislation in certain situations imply terms into that contract.

- In the event of a dispute in the terms of the contract or the employer varies the terms of the contract, the doctor should seek advice from their trade union body or a specialist employment adviser. If you continue to work for more than a reasonable period without objection, then acquiescence is construed as acceptance of the contract.

Chapter 2
THE DOCTOR AND THE PATIENT

DUTY OF CARE *(love thy neighbour!)*

In this chapter, the notion of duty of care will be examined , who owes it, to whom it is owed and consider the legal tests for duty.

General Principles of the Duty of Care:

The duty of care defines the interests that are protected by the tort of negligence marking out the boundaries of what is or is not actionable. The biblical commandment that you are to love your neighbour as yourself is the bedrock of the duty of care. It modifies our behaviour to give thought and caution to our 'neighbour' – persons who are in the area of foreseeable danger. A duty of care in certain circumstances, imposes an obligation to exercise reasonable care to avoid acts or omissions which can be reasonably foreseen to be likely to cause physical harm to persons or property. Where there is no duty to exercise care then there is no legal consequence.

Negligence is the failure to exercise that care. It may consist in omitting to do something which ought to be done or in doing something which ought to be done either in a different manner or not at all. The considerations in establishing negligence are the absence of care which has caused damage, with a demonstrable relation of cause and effect between the two. The law of negligence has been developed and refined by the common law. An important case which is regarded as landmark in the tort of negligence is *Donoghue and Stevenson [1932] AC 562*. The House of Lords held that the manufacturer of ginger beer could be liable in negligence for injury to an ultimate consumer of the product as a result of its defective condition (the remains of a decomposed snail in the bottle, the consumption of which caused the plaintiff's illness)

Lord Atkin in his judgement in the case said: 'You must take reasonable care to avoid acts or omissions which you can reasonably foresee would likely to injure your neighbour'. He created what is known as the 'neighbour test' and went on to define your neighbour as persons 'who are so closely and directly affected by my act that I ought reasonably to have them in contemplation as being so affected when I am directing my mind to the acts or omissions which are called in question'. As a general rule, there is little doubt that a person has a duty not to cause damage either to people or property by some positive action or omission.

In the doctor- patient relationship, a prima facie duty of care arises because the parties are in sufficient relationship of proximity as to be regarded as neighbours such that, in the reasonable contemplation of the doctor, carelessness on his part may be likely to cause damage to the patient.

Legal test for Duty:

The test, then, is reasonable foresight of harm to persons whom it is foreseeable are likely to be harmed by my carelessness.

The formal requirements that must be satisfied for a duty of care to exist are:

a. Foreseeability of damage- the more foreseeable the harm, the more likely a court will be to hold that the there is a duty of care.

b. A sufficiently 'proximate' relationship between the parties as between a doctor and his patient.

c. It must be 'just and reasonable' to impose a duty. This reduces or limits the scope of duty to your neighbour – Pharisees and Samaritans alike and that for every mischance in an accident prone world someone solvent must be liable in damages. As per Lord Bridge in *Caparo and Dickman [1990] 1All ER 568*

From the above it can be seen that there is an intricate interrelationship between the 3 limbs of the test- the more foreseeable the harm , the more likely a court will be to hold that the relationship is proximate and likely that it is just and reasonable to impose a duty.

The doctor patient relationship crystallises into a legal relationship when a request for medical services by an individual is reciprocated by a consequent undertaking by the doctor to provide services. Arising out of this request and undertaking, the law creates the doctor / patient relationship – a proximate relationship as to make them 'neighbours'.

'Proximity requires such a relationship between the parties as renders it fair, just and reasonable that liability must be imposed ....' *Ward J. in Ravenscroft- v- Rederiaktiebolaget Transatlantic [1991] 3 All ER 73, 84-5.*

The legal effect of this relationship is that the doctor owes the patient a duty of care. There is now a sufficiently proximate relationship to be careful not to cause foreseeable damage. The medical man's duty of care arises independently of any contract with his patient. It is based upon the fact that the medical man has undertaken the care and treatment of the patient.

Duty arising from professional obligation

The General Medical Council (GMC) regulates and licenses the practice of doctors in U.K under the provisions of the Medical Practice Act 1983. Its objective is to make sure that the public is served by doctors who have the qualities it expects and to protect the public from doctors whose conduct , professional performance or health places patients at risk. In line with this aim, it sets general standards of professional competence and conduct. The GMC sets professionally led medical regulation by setting out the principles of Good Medical Practice- at the core of which it lists the duties of a doctor. It links these principles and duties, which command widespread public support , explicitly to a doctor's registration. This forms the basis of the professional obligation between the doctor and the patient.

Doctors registering with the GMC are therefore making a commitment and implied professional obligation to their patients and to their profession to practice accordingly. The GMC handbook – *Good Medical Practice (2001)* sets the framework of professional standard within which doctors must practice in the U.K. On registration with the GMC there is an express duty of care imposed on doctors. These duties are stated in broad terms in the handbook referred to above.

From the above foregoing a doctor owes a duty of care to his patient in the normal course of events to act with reasonable skill and care.

Implied duty arising from the contract.

Hospital doctors have a legal relationship with the employing NHS Trust or Primary Care Trust (PCT) under a contract of service. It is an implied term of a contract of employment that the employee will exercise reasonable care and skill in the performance of their duties. This will apply as well to doctors. A doctor will be in breach of this duty if he performs his duties carelessly or incompetently and may also be liable to indemnify the employer for any loss suffered by the employer by reason of the breach. This implied contractual duty is applicable to doctors in the NHS Trust or PCT.

The common law draws an important distinction between treatment under the NHS and private treatment. Where services are provided pursuant to a statutory obligation there is no contractual relationship. This will be the case for NHS hospital and GP services. Liability for most clinical negligence claims is under the law of Negligence. However in the case of private patients there will be a contractual relationship between the parties. The contract is between the patient and the doctor and not the patient and private hospital. This gives private patients an additional claim in breach of contract against the doctor directly as well as negligence. The implication of this really is in the time limits for commencing legal action- up to six years in a breach of contract claim and up to three years in a negligence claim.

Implied by Legislation

Legislation in the form of an Act of Parliament or delegated legislation in the form of Statutory Instruments have developed and established a duty of care in certain circumstances as follows:

- The supply of Goods and Services Act 1982: It is implied into a contract under which a person (the supplier) agrees to carry out a service, a duty to perform the service with reasonable care and skill (section 13). This implied duty will apply as between a doctor and his patient in the course of duty. In the course of duty will include acting as a rescuer in an emergency outside the usual place of work.

- Consumer Protection Act 1987 : This imposes a strict liability on the producers or suppliers of defective goods. This will apply to defective drugs, appliances and prosthesis. There is no need to prove negligence. The supplier can become liable if he cannot identify the producer. Doctors who give their patients' drugs or appliances from the consulting room will become suppliers under the Act. It follows that they must be able to identify the producer of a drug or medical product if required failing which could be liable in a subsequent litigation. Drugs, appliances and prosthesis supplied from the hospital will make the Trust a supplier. It is particularly important when giving out medicinal products and devices to document clearly the name of the drug, its source- the manufacturer, batch number and expiry date. It is now common practice where a prosthesis, device or implant is inserted in a patient, to attach the product identification label to the patient's notes. Patients may sue under the Act for up to 10 years hence records will need to be preserved for that length of time. Some areas of clinical practice where this is relevant is as follows:
    - Obstetrics & Gynaecology - Insertion of intrauterine contraceptive device, insertion of Oestrogen and testosterone implants
    - Orthopaedic Surgery : Artificial joints, fixation screws and plates
    - General Surgery : Breast implants, ureteric stents.

- European Convention on Human Rights 1950 (ECHR)
  Human Rights Act 1998
  In the context of duty and negligence Art 2 of the ECHR is the likely area of a claim. The Article provided for a right to life which can be construed to mean that it positively provided for a certain quality of life. Claims may be brought for not receiving medical treatment for a

life threatening condition, not receiving different and better (probably more expensive) treatment, not receiving specific non-life threatening treatment e.g. IVF.

Fiduciary duty

A fiduciary relationship is one held or given in trust. It exists where a person has placed a confidence in another person, whereby that person, having been privy to such information is under a duty not to disclose information gained from such relationship or act in a way to breach trust and confidence. Doctors are in a fiduciary relationship with their patients' and have an overriding responsibility towards their patient dependent on public confidence. They are under a duty to act in good faith towards their patients who are in the position of reliance on them. This is the bedrock of the duty of confidence as between a doctor and his patient. A facet of the fiduciary duty is the rule that a doctor must not place himself in a position where his personal interest and his duties towards his patients' come into 'conflict'.

Conflict of interest can arise in a number of contexts. Some are obvious e.g most doctor would identify that an offer of payment to refer patients to a private clinic raises issues of conflict. An example of conflict arising is an expert witness who writes a report to the courts on a past or present patient. Whilst the overriding duty to the court is paramount, there is clearly a conflict of interest in his duty to the courts and to the patient. Conflict arises also where a doctor buys or sells goods from his patient or receives generous gifts or advantages from the patient.

The GMC provides some guidance on this in Good Medical Practice (2001) reminding doctors that they 'must not ask for or accept any inducement, gift or hospitality ' which may affect or be seen to affect their judgement. (para 55)

Another area of conflict relates to sponsorship of conferences and meetings. While it is normal practice for medical journals to require authors of papers to declare any competing interests, this practice is often not followed at medical meetings and conferences. Delegates are therefore uninformed of who is paying the speaker and whether their contributions might be influenced by such payments or other sponsorship and benefits. The GMC Standards and Ethics Committee has agreed that where a contributor to an educational meeting has been sponsored by a pharmaceutical company that this should be announced at the beginning of the meeting, with information about whether the speaker will be discussing products manufactured by the sponsoring company. This will inform the delegates of who is paying the speaker and whether their contributions might be influenced by such payments or other sponsorship or benefits. (GMC News Issue 2, June 2005 pg 15)

Many GPs are increasingly involved in the referral of patients to the private sector or where a patient transfers from the NHS to Private care and vice versa. Referral must be made after consideration of the clinical needs of the patient and must be made to the organisation or institution the doctor feels is most appropriate in the particular case. It is therefore unacceptable to accept inducements to refer patients to particular health care facilities or fast track your private patient to your NHS care as this is likely to compromise the doctor's independent judgement. If you have a financial interest in an organisation to which you plan to refer a patient, you must tell the patient about your interest. (Duties of a doctor : Good Medical Practice (2001) para 53-58). Similarly in prescribing drugs the decision must be based on the medical needs and interest of the patient. A doctor must not allow his decision to be fettered by pharmaceutical companies through financial incentives.

As regards gifts and promotional activities, you should not ask for or accept any material rewards, except those of insignificant value, from companies that sell or market drugs or appliances. You must not ask for or accept fees for agreeing to meet sales representatives. You may accept personal travel grants and hospitality from companies for conferences or educational meetings, as long as the main purpose of the event is educational. The amount you receive must not be more than you would normally spend if you were paying for yourself.

Duty to a third party

The concept of duty of care can be extended to third parties who in particular circumstances may be in potential danger and in a relationship with the patient as being so closely and directly affected by treatment or advice that the doctor ought to have them in mind. This thereby requires the doctor to take reasonable steps to avoid foreseeable damage. A doctor does not have control over the conduct of patients but in exceptional circumstances injury to a third party is within the reasonable contemplation of the parties to give rise to a duty to take reasonable precautions to avoid it. An epileptic patient should be warned to avoid certain activities e.g. driving and high impact sports. If the doctor fails to so warn and a third party is injured in an accident involving the patient, the doctor would be responsible both to the patient and the third party.

This duty to third parties is particularly important in patients who are at risk to physically injure another in Mental Health Units. In *Holgarth -v- Lancashire Mental Hospital Board [1937]* the defendants were held liable in negligence where a patient was let out and assaulted the claimant. If a patient makes genuine threats of serious injury to an identified third party and there was a real risk that the threats would be carried out, the doctor will owe a duty of care to the potential victim. The duty will arise from the defendant's knowledge of the foreseeable damage of serious physical harm to the third party.

In *Pittman Estate -v- Bain (1994) 112 DLR 4th 257, a G.P* was held liable for failing to inform his patient that there was a high risk that he was HIV positive, as a result of which the patient's spouse also contracted HIV. It may be reasoned that this is contrary to the duty of confidentiality to the patient. This duty is not an absolute duty if disclosure in public interest outweighs the duty of confidentiality to the patient. You may disclose information about a patient whether living or dead in order to protect a third party from the risk of death or serious harm.

For example you may disclose information to a known sexual contact of a patient with HIV where you have reason to think that the patient has not informed that person and cannot be persuaded to do so. In such circumstances you should tell the patient before you make the disclosure and must be prepared to justify the decision to disclose to a third party. (GMC: 'Serious Communicable Diseases' para 22)

Another example of the remit of duty to a third party is in cases of nervous shock. It is now well established that a person who has negligently killed or injured A or put A in peril of injury or death may be liable to B for a psychiatric injury resulting from the perception of the events. Such third parties are defined legally as 'secondary victims' and must have a sufficiently close relationship of emotional tie with the injured victim. A parent or spouse of the injured victim would be more readily accepted as a person likely to be affected and accordingly within the range of a duty of care owed by the defendant. The term nervous shock is a medically recognised psychiatric illness or disorder arising in these circumstances. In *Herican-v- Ruan [1991] 3All ER 65* it was held that a claimant who had identified his son's body at the mortuary was entitled to succeed for psychological trauma following the death, although he was not present at the scene of the accident or the aftermath.

Similarly in *Walters –v- North Glamorgan NHS Trust [2002] EWHC 321 (QB), [2002] All ER (D) 65* the mother of a baby claimed psychiatric injury as a result of witnessing her child's decline and death due to misdiagnosis at the hospital.

Duty to the Fetus & Embryo

The fetus and the embryo come within the group of third parties within the proximity of the doctors care as to take reasonable steps to avoid foreseeable harm. Though the fetus and embryo lack legal status, the law still provides protection from harm especially in the realm of medical treatments.

The statutory duty of care owed to the embryo is enshrined in the Congenital Disabilities (Civil Liability) Act 1976 . This Act grants a right of action to a child who is born alive and disabled in respect of the disability if it is caused by an occurrence which affected either parents ability to have a normal healthy child or affected the mother during her pregnancy or so affected her or the child in the course of its birth, so that the child is born with disabilities which would not otherwise have been present.(s1(2)a)(b). The Act covers negligence in the course of the selection or handling of an embryo or gametes in Assisted Conception Techniques. Similarly any medical treatment which affects a man in his ability to have a normal healthy child, or affects a woman in that or so affects her when she is pregnant that her child is born with disabilities which would not otherwise have been present is actionable under the Act. This would include preconception treatment such as radiotherapy and chemotherapy.

In *Reay-v- BNF; Hope- v- BNF Plc [1994] 5Med LR1*, the claimant alleged that paternal preconception irradiation caused mutation in their father's sperm which in turn caused predisposition to leukaemia and or non-hodgkins lymphoma in the next generation. Though the claim failed on the element of causation.(causal link between the breach and the damage)the judge did say that the courts did not have a problem in finding that the defendants had a legal duty. If the damage caused was foreseeable then a possible breach of duty is likely to be found.

In the case of a preconceptual occurrence affecting the parents ability to have a normal healthy child, the doctor is not liable to the child if either or both the parents knew the risk of disability (s1(14)). This derivative duty to the child crystallises from the doctor's duty to the parents except that it is not necessary to show that the parent suffered any injury hence avoiding any argument that a damaged child cannot sue because the mother did not suffer harm.

SPECIFIC DUTIES OF THE DOCTOR

The doctor's duty of care is a single duty encompassing advice, diagnosis, treatment, follow-up and referral as appropriate. This single indivisible duty was confirmed in the case of *Sidaway-v- Board of Governors of the Bethlehem Royal Hospitals [1985] AC 871* by Lord Diplock (pg 895)...... the doctor's relationship with his patient which gives rise to the normal duty of care to exercise his skill and judgement to improve the patient's health …..has hitherto been treated as a single comprehensive duty. This general duty is not subject to dissection into a number of component parts to which different criteria apply.'

The undertaking a doctor gives to a patient is to attend, take a full history from the patient, carry out an appropriate physical examination and where necessary diagnostic tests. The diagnosis must be reviewed regularly and if necessary appropriate referral to another specialist should be initiated. The advice to the patient can include reassurance, alternative care and a range of treatment options. With this in mind the scope for a clinical negligence claim is diverse and varied.

- Duty to attend
  A failure to attend to the patient promptly or not at all may be deemed negligent if a reasonable doctor would have attended in the circumstance. In Barnett -v- Chelsea and Kensington Hospital

Management Committee [1968] 1 All ER 1068, three watchmen attended the hospital feeling unwell. The nurse telephoned the casualty officer who did not see the men, but said they should go home and see their family doctor. One of the men died five hours later. Nield J held that in these circumstances the casualty officer should have seen and examined the deceased and was negligent in failing to do so. By giving advice over the phone the doctor had clearly instituted care of the three watchmen though inadequately. The liability will depend on the seriousness of the patient's condition, the information given and the competing needs of other patients at the time.. The latter factor is particularly relevant where doctors are on cover for various units of the same speciality and are inundated with calls from these units. This often leads to delays in responding to calls to see patients which can have serious consequences.

In *Bolitho-v- City and Hackney Health Authority [1993] 4 Med. LR 381* the defendant's doctors who failed to respond to an emergency bleep call for assistance by a nurse on a paediatric ward were found negligent.

- Duty to take a medical history
  Listening to the patients' history is as much a part of the art of medicine as clinical examination. Modern aids to diagnosis no doubt assist the medical practitioner in varying degrees depending on the circumstances. They can hardly take the place of listening to the patients' symptoms. Medical evidence indicates that a significant number of clinical diagnoses can be determined from a comprehensive medical history and a thorough physical examination. The duty to take a history requires the doctor to listen to what the patient is saying. Inattention to the symptoms of the patient can effect on the diagnosis and treatment of a patient resulting in substandard or inappropriate care amounting to negligence.
  A patient should be given sufficient time to describe the symptoms and an opportunity to ask questions. Inadequate time for consultation which is a recurrent problem at consultation is not a defence if substandard care results.
  Case scenarios
    - A doctor did not make an enquiry into the patient's medical history for allergies before administering an injection of Penicillin. The patient died

from an allergic reaction to the drug. The doctor was aware of the remote possibility of danger, but nervertheless carried on with his normal practice of not making any enquiry because he had not had any mishaps before.

- *A patient was referred for an Intravenous Urogram (IVU) for back pain. The doctor had not taken an adequate history nor carried out less invasive testing such as an ultrasound. The patient died from an allergic reaction to the contrast dye used in the IVU. Sadly the deceased never had any symptoms or signs relevant to the urinary tract.*

- *An 89year old lady suffered intractable bladder pain due to interstitial cystitis. At an outpatient follow up the Gynaecology Registrar, failed to take an adequate history from the patient and made a decision based on the referral letter which stated that the patient was incontinent. The patient was prescribed catheterisation which worsened the symptoms and was clearly the wrong line of management.*

- Duty to examine

    There is much to say that the simplest invaluable diagnostic tool for the physician is a comprehensive and relevant physical examination. The outcome of this enables appropriate investigations to be arranged to confirm or refute a diagnosis.

    Case Scenario

    - *A general practitioner failed to examine a lady with an abdominal mass where sufficient indication of fetal parts would have aroused the GP's suspicion and he should have referred to the antenatal clinic rather than a gynaecology outpatient department. The patient was 32 weeks pregnant and had a preterm delivery whilst waiting in the emergency department.*

    - *A General Practitioner failed to examine a patient's breasts for lumps following an inconclusive Ultrasound scan, thus missing the opportunity to confirm or revise his provisional diagnosis.*

    - *A gynaecology registrar failed to perform a pelvic examination on a lady presenting with postmenopausal bleeding. The lady was sent for an ultrasound scan of the pelvis which was normal. She continued to bleed and an examination under anaesthesia was performed. A fungating carcinoma of the cervix involving the lateral vaginal wall was found.*

- Duty to diagnose

    Following history taking and examination of the patient, the doctor must consider a differential of diagnoses including one of no abnormality. The diagnosis will be judged on all the available facts when a diagnosis was given or not given, not at a future date with the benefit of sharper vision and hindsight.

    The doctor should review the diagnosis and be ready with an alternative theory to direct treatment if the patient does not improve. Where a potentially life threatening condition is included in a differential diagnosis, there is a duty on the physician to take prompt steps to confirm or rule it out with reasonable dispatch. Failure to arrange appropriate tests can be held to be negligent if a reasonable doctor would have arranged those tests.

    Caselaw is rife with examples of error of diagnosis. In *Elder –v- Greenwich & Deptford Hospital Management Committee, The Times March 7 1984* the failure of a hospital casualty doctor to diagnose appendicitis in a child who presented with pain on the right side of the abdomen and vomiting was held to be negligent. In *Hotson-v- East Berkshire Area Health Authority [1987] 2All ER 909* the failure to identify a dislocated fracture of the neck apparent on x-ray was held to be negligent.

    Case scenario:

    − An afro carribean lady was scheduled to undergo surgery for a knee operation. The Anaesthetist failed to ensure that a sickle test was performed prior to surgery. The patient suffered a sickle crisis during the operation because of inadequate oxygenation.

    − A patient had a previous obstetric trauma with difficulty in the delivery of the shoulders (shoulder dystocia) of the infant weighing 4.2 kg. In the next pregnancy she was not screened for gestational diabetes nor an ultrasound arranged for an estimation of the fetal weight late in pregnancy. At delivery she had another traumatic delivery with a neonatal death.

Fear of being found negligent for failing to use appropriate diagnostic tests has increased defensive practices in the form of unnecessary testing. If a diagnostic test or procedure is deemed unnecessary according to the standards of a reasonably competent doctor then it will be negligent to perform it and moreso if the patient suffers damage. This was the thrust of the claim in *Maynard –v- West Midlands Regional Health Authority [1984] WLR 634*. The defendant doctor had performed a diagnostic operation which resulted in damage to the claimant.

The Royal College of Radiologists and the National Radiological Protection Board have estimated that unnecessary x-rays cause between 100-25- deaths/year. Poor management, excessive dosage and unnecessary repeat x-rays are blamed. It is estimated that a fifth of radiological examinations carried out in NHS hospitals are clinically unhelpful, undertaken for the purpose of avoiding litigation and at a cost of £50million per annum. It can only be a matter of time before 'unnecessary' exposure to investigative tests becomes a cause for claim in its own right.

- Duty to follow up test results

  Where a doctor has performed or requested an investigation, there is a duty to follow up the test result, act on it appropriately and inform the patient of the result. Wrongly interpreting test results or failing to notify another health professional who needs to know to institute treatment or the patient personally may be held to be negligent. In *Holmes –v- Board of Hospital Trustees of the City of London (1977) 81 DLR* the doctors responsible for the plaintiff's treatment ordered x-rays to be carried out but delayed for 5 days before examining them. They were held negligent for failing to inform themselves of the factual data which they had identified was necessary to the plaintiff's diagnosis and which they knew or ought to have known was available.

  In *McKay-v- Essex AHA [1982] QB 1166* the claimant argued that the doctor who had taken blood samples for rubella immunity tests failed to inform the mother that she and the unborn baby were infected with rubella. Consequently the claimant child was born with severe disabilities. The claim failed but it was however held to be negligent in failing to follow up the test results.

- Duty to refer to another specialist

  1 A doctor must constantly review the original diagnosis in the face of the patient's symptoms not improving or new available information in

the form of test results. This duty extends to post operative conditions the patient may develop. Where a doctor is unable to diagnose or treat the patient then he should seek advice from a specialist or refer to one. It can be held negligent for failing to spot something serious that the patient ought to have been sent for further tests or referred to a specialist who is capable of making the diagnosis. If the doctor attempts to treat the patient himself, he is in effect, undertaking work beyond his competence, for which he will be held liable if harm results.

Case Scenario

- A surgeon made a *diagnosis of Pelvic inflammatory disease in a female patient and referred to the Gynaecologist who confirmed the diagnosis. The patient whilst under the care of the Gynaecologist failed to respond to intravenous antibiotics for 48hrs. She died from peritonitis due to a ruptured appendix. Whilst the wrong diagnosis in itself is not negligent, failing to take account of the non improvement of the patient's symptom and referring back to the surgical team is.*

- *A patient presented with symptoms of fever, sweating and shivering to the G.P who diagnosed influenza. The patient subsequently died from malaria, having recently returned from Uganda. General Practitioners do not commonly come across malaria, but in the circumstances it should have entered the G.P's mind that a tropical disease is a possibility. He should have been alerted to the probability that it might not be an indigenous disease.*

SUMMARY

- The doctor's relationship with his patient gives rise to the normal duty of care to exercise reasonable care, skill and judgement.
- The legal duty of care is a single duty encompassing a duty to see, a duty to diagnose, a duty to treat, a duty to refer etc.
- The legal duty is owed irrespective of the experience of the doctor.
- In certain circumstances, a legal duty may be directly owed by the doctor to a third party.
- Doctors working for the NHS, a public authority may owe additional duties to their patients under the Human Rights Act 1998 and the European Convention on Human Rights 1950.

STANDARD OF CARE

This chapter will examine and critique the legal rules used by the courts to determine the difficult question as to whether the treatment of a patient amounted to negligent treatment. The discussion of breach will involve determination of two questions:
a. the legal determination of the standard of care
b. how the courts determine the factual question of whether the defendant has breached that standard on the facts of the case.

Standard of care is concerned with whether the doctor's conduct can be characterised as careless. It involves an assessment by the court of how, in the circumstances the doctor ought to have behaved. This is a question of law for the courts guided by the doctor's peers. A doctor will be judged against the standard of his peers in the particular field of practice. 'Like is compared with like'. The test is the standard of the ordinary skilled man exercising and professing to have that special skill. A man need not possess the highest experience and skill at the risk of being found negligent.

The standard of care applicable to the medical profession is that stated by McNair in Bolam –v- Friern Health Management Committee [1957] 1 WLR 582 pp 587 now commonly known as the Bolam test : A doctor is not guilty of negligence if he has acted in accordance with a practice accepted as proper by a responsible body of medical men skilled in that particular art. This standard applies to all aspects of a doctors duty towards his or her patient. In the field of medical negligence, the Bolam test is now recognised as almost determinative of what the claimant must show to establish negligence on the part of the defendant.

The test is in two limbs;
– What is the standard; and
– On the facts of the case, whether the defendant's conduct fell below that standard.

The facts of the Bolam case:
The claimant was given electroconvulsive therapy and as a result of this treatment sustained fractures. He argued that the doctor was negligent in not giving him relaxant drugs (which admittedly would have excluded the risk of fractures). Secondly if relaxant drugs were not used in failing to restrain him manually. Finally in not warning him of the risks involved in the treatment.

There were different opinions in the medical field as to whether the claimant should have been given relaxant drugs and whether the claimant should have been so warned. The defendant doctor was found not negligent because he was able to show that he acted in accordance with the accepted medical practice of his peers.

Negligence is a departure from practice which in fact are actually adopted by the profession. Alternatively negligence may be a departure from standards that ought to be adopted by the profession (whether or not they are adopted). Conversely, the fact that the defendant has departed from common practice is not necessarily negligent either. It may be prima facie evidence of negligence but it is not conclusive. The standard is described as one 'accepted as proper by a responsible body of opinion'. Despite the authority with which the Bolam test has been imbued, the courts may condemn a common professional practice as unreasonable and therefore negligent. This means that the courts can consider a practice as irresponsible. In *Bolitho-v- City & Hackney HA [1997] 4 All ER 771*, the Bolam approach was re-examined to see if it was still appropriate and whether the Courts will be more willing to criticise commonly accepted professional medical practice.

Lord Browne Wilkinson said 'In the vast majority of cases the fact that distinguished experts in the field are of a particular opinion will demonstrate the reasonableness of that opinion........ . But if in rare cases, it can be demonstrated that professional opinion is not capable of withstanding logical analysis, the judge is entitled to hold that the body of opinion is not reasonable or responsible'.

The doors having been opened by Lord Browne Wilkinson will give more scope for a claimant to challenge the views of a respectable body of medical opinion in relation to diagnosis and treatment. It is highly likely that more claimants will try to cast doubt on the acceptability of professional medical evidence by arguing that their position does not stand up to logical analysis. What has emerged from the Bolitho case are as follows -

a. that the principle laid down in Bolam still apply. The House of Lords is quite clear in its belief that the courts should only rarely impose its own view as to what is reasonable medical practice in particular situations.

b. where there is doubt as to whether the body of medical opinion used to support the action is 'responsible, reasonable and respectable' a judge may choose to find that the defendants action were not justified.

c. in determining whether a body of medical opinion is 'responsible, reasonable and respectable' the courts should be satisfied that those experts have properly considered the comparative risks and benefit to reach a defensible conclusion.

d. What is reasonable is a question of law to be determined by the court, who place heavy reliance on expert evidence. In the vast majority of cases, evidence of distinguished experts in the field will be conclusive to support a defendant's case.

Levels of Skill

The defendant is not to be judged by the standards of the most experienced or the most skilful, nor by the standards of the least qualified and experienced.

In accordance with Bolam, the standard is that of the ordinary competent practitioner in the defendant's field of Medicine. The standard of care is judged by reference to the status of the defendant and not to his personality or experience. No allowance is made for the personal idiosyncrasies, physical or mental illness of the defendant. The defendant must come up to the standard of the speciality.

The differing grades of hospital doctors and specialisation can make it difficult to prove a single standard of care. Adopting differing standards based on the experience and qualification is too uncertain and subjective. It will leave an arduous task for the court of specifying a subjective level of competence for each defendant. This would mean that for the patient the standard of care received would depend on who is on duty when care was given. Against the differing standards rule, Mustill LJ in *Wilsher – Essex HA [1987] QB 730; CA[1988] AC 1074 HL* expounded the judicial response to the standard of care applied in complex professional scenarios with a number of medical professionals with differing designations, tasks and abilities.

Facts of the case:

Martin Wilsher was born prematurely and was suffering from a number of illnesses. He was placed in a special care baby unit at the hospital. While he was in the unit a catheter was twice inserted in a vein rather than an artery and on both occasions he was given excess oxygen. The medical team in the unit consisted of a senior Registrar (SR), two consultants, several senior house officers and trained nurses. The doctor administering the oxygen was a junior and inexperienced. He asked the SR to check that that the correct procedure had been undertaken but the SR failed to spot the mistake. The baby was subsequently found to be suffering from retrolental fibroplasia which causes blindness.

'.....this notion of a duty tailored to the actor rather than to the act which he elects to perform, has no place in the law of tort......Public hospital medicine has always been organised so that young doctors and nurses learn on the job.....the longer term interests of patients as a whole are best served by maintaining the present system, even if this may diminish the legal rights of the individual patient for afterall medicine is about curing not litigation'. (LJ Mustill)

In the Court of Appeal, it was agreed that the standard of care expected of the junior doctor was not the same as that of the experienced counterpart. The majority of the Court of Appeal dismissed this argument and applied the Bolam test. Glidewell, J commenting said that if there was not a uniform standard of care then.........inexperience would frequently be argued as a defence to an action for professional negligence.' The harshness of this comment was eased by Glidewell LJ's acknowledgement that the junior doctor who consults a superior for advice will have come up to the standard expected. The standard of care to be expected of the junior doctor in *Wilsher -v- Essex AHA* was regarded by the Court of Appeal as the standard of the reasonable junior doctor acting in the Special Care Baby Unit. This case went on further to analyse the standard of care in an emergency situation. Mustill LJ stated : ' An emergency may overburden the available resources, and, if an individual is forced by circumstances to do many things at once, the fact that he does one of them incorrectly should not lightly be taken as negligence'

Patients should be able to expect a minimum standard of expertise in a particular area and should also recognise the reality that experience is often best obtained on the job itself. The burden of this test seems prejudicial on the doctors who are seeking to train in a speciality. This threat to the doctors posed by such a standard has lead to certain specialities being unpopular for training and lead to defensive practices. The difficulty for junior /inexperienced doctors is that their very lack of experience may prevent them from knowing when they are out of their depth. Nonetheless they will be held negligent for failing to refer patients to more senior colleagues or another specialist.

In *Payne-v- St Helier Group HMCC (1952)* a patient had been kicked in the stomach by a horse and subsequently died from peritonitis. A casualty officer was held to be negligent for failing to detain the patient for examination by a doctor of consultant rank.

The above two rulings have implications for clinical practice: Junior doctors for fear of litigation, will refer to a senior colleague or another Specialist. This may unduly delay treatment, increase inappropriate referrals and inundate senior colleagues with 'nuisance' enquiries.

Junior doctors within the NHS are often overworked and stretched to the limit of their endurance and professional capacity or placed under onerous tasks and responsibilities. The hospital could be made directly liable for placing the junior doctor in a position with which he was not qualified to do. A health authority which so conducts its hospital that it fails to provide doctors of sufficient skill and experience to give the treatment offered at the hospital may be directly liable in negligence to the patient.

It is well known that junior doctors work under immense pressure that may impair their performance significantly and often fail to seek help from more senior colleagues early. Faced with this scenario, the doctor must act in the best interest of the patient. 'You must recognise the limits of your professional competence; If you know that … your judgement or performance could be significantly affected …..you must take and follow advice from a consultant in occupational health or another suitably qualified colleague on whether, and in what ways you should modify your practice' (GMC: Good Medical Practice 2001 para 3, 59).

Therefore seek help early rather than soldier it alone. You will be more unpopular if harm occurs to a patient.

SUMMARY

- The standard of care is that which is accepted as proper by a responsible body of medical men in the speciality.
- The standard of care depends on the post occupied by the doctor and not on the level of training the doctor has received.
- Whilst recognising the real pressures of training on the job and the existence of emergency situations the junior doctor must meet the standard of care expected of his status. Inexperience is no defence.
- The junior doctor will not be liable if he seeks senior advice. Liability will then fall on the senior colleague for lack of supervision.
- A specialist must exercise the standard of care of a reasonably competent specialist in his field. To date the courts have been reluctant from demanding a higher standard of care from a specialist.
- If a doctor undertakes a clinical task, holding himself out as possessing the skills and knowledge, it can be assumed that he has the competence to perform the task with due care and skill. If he exceeds that expertise it will constitute a breach of the standard of care.
- The standard of care required may be lower in an emergency.

'ACCEPTED PRACTICE'

The second limb in the determination of the standard of care is how the courts determine the factual question of whether the defendant has breached that standard on the facts of the case.

The Bolam test expects that the defendant doctor acts in accordance with accepted practice. Accepted practice means a practice accepted as proper by the defendant's peers. They are in substance formalised accepted practice and it is therefore not surprising that conduct which departs from that may incur liability. General and approved practice need not be universal but must be approved of and adhered to by a substantial number of reputable practitioners holding the relevant specialist or general qualifications. The fact that one particular expert, however eminent adopts a particular practice does not mean that the practice becomes an acceptable body of opinion affording protection to a professional following it.

The test is one of acceptable and responsible practice. The use of the adjectives- responsible, reasonable and respectable all show that the court has to be satisfied that the exponents of the body of opinion relied on can demonstrate that such opinion has a logical basis.

'In particular where it involves weighing of risks versus benefits, the judge before accepting a body of opinion as being responsible, reasonable or respectable, will need to be satisfied that, in forming their views, the experts have directed their minds to the question of comparative risks and benefit and have reached a defensible conclusion on the matter.' Lord Brown-Wilkinson *in Bolitho-v- City of Hackney HA 1997 4 All ER 778* .

To assist and inform the courts in this task, the expert witness is requested to give an opinion. The question of quality of the practice remains and it applies where the bodies of opinion are of equal competence. The protection which adherence to accepted professional practice provides though extensive is not absolute. Following a common practice is only evidence of having satisfied the standard of reasonable care, however, it is not conclusive, since the court may find that the practice itself is negligent.

This was the decision of the courts in the case of *Hucks-v- Cole [1994] Med LR 393,CA.*

Facts of the case:

he Mrs Hucks had recently given birth and developed puerperal fever which was rare in the 1960's. The GP had failed to treat Mrs Hucks with Penicillin as a result she developed septicaemia. The defendant said he acted in accordance with the reasonable practice of other doctors with obstetric experience. This defence was rejected. The doctor should have taken the requisite steps when he could see that the absence of treatment posed a serious risk to the woman's health.

Sachs LJ said 'where the evidence shows that a lacuna in professional practice exists by which the risks of grave danger are knowingly undertaken, then, however small the risks, the courts must anxiously examine that lacuna, particularly if the risks can be easily and inexpensively avoided. If the court, finds on analysis of the reasons given for not taking those precautions that, in the light of current professional knowledge, there is no proper basis for the lacuna and that it is definitely not reasonable that those risks should have been taken, its function is to state that fact and where necessary to state that it constitutes negligence.'

The judge added that the fact that other practitioners would have done the same as the defendant is a 'very weighty matter to be put into the scale ...... but it was not decisive'.

Similarly the court ruled against accepted medical practice in *Newell and Newell-v- Goldenberg (1995)* and held that the defendant was negligent in failing to warn of the risks of failure of a vasectomy. The body of medical opinion was neither responsible nor reasonable.

The court has to be satisfied that the experts of a body of opinion can demonstrate a logical basis for the opinion.

GUIDELINES & PROTOCOLS

The judicial concept of accepted practice introduces the subject of guidelines, protocols and integrated care pathways in clinical practice. Nearly all areas of medical practice have seen the deluge of pro-formas, protocols and guidelines. Their objectives are to reduce the variations in clinical care and maintain consistent high quality clinical care. Many of these have their origin from professional/regulatory bodies (GMC, BMA, RCOG, RCS) government organisations (NICE, HFEA, CHAI) and

Hospital Guideline Development Groups.

Guidelines and protocols are systematically developed statements to assist practitioners about appropriate healthcare for specific clinical circumstances, setting out standards of care or safe working practices and procedures. They are the backbone of multidisciplinary care giving guidance to several practitioners involved in the care of a patient. They are in substance no more than formalised accepted practice and it is therefore not surprising that conduct which departs from the 'code of practice' may lead to liability. They may constitute significant evidence of what is a reasonable standard of care.

What is the legal status of guidelines and protocols?
Clinical guidelines have a supportive role to expert witness testimony in determining the standard of care in medical litigation. The judicial response is drawn from the comments of Lord Woolf J. in *Lloyd Cheyham & Co Ltd -v- Littlejohn & Co Ltd (1985) 2PN 154*. 'As to the proper treatment of such statements......while they are not conclusive, so that a departure from their terms necessarily involves a breach of a duty of care, and they are not as the explanatory foreword makes clear, rigid rules, they are very strong evidence as to what is the proper standard which should be adopted and unless there is some justification, a departure from this will be regarded as constituting a breach of duty'.

In legal proceedings, guidelines and protocols are proof to evidence a professional standard. The courts are assisted and influenced by these statements in setting the legal standard of care. Clearly the authority for those statements will be weighted to (governmental or professional bodies) and evidence of scientific validation. NICE guidelines for example will carry significant weight in legal proceedings as they provide a benchmark of the standard of care and are supported by government policy. Trusts therefore have an obligation to ensure that the implementation of NICE guidelines is facilitated through their clinical governance agenda. Hence whilst they do not have the force of the law i.e legally binding, the courts and expert witnesses will refer to them in establishing what is current and accepted practice.

The court has to be satisfied that 'accepted practice' has a logical basis for its approach. A 'logical basis' must demonstrate that it is based on evidence from good quality research which is validated for quality control. Trusts will need to take cognisance of this in their risk management strategy in the development and implementation of local guidelines to ensure that they use high level evidence and are updated at regular intervals. The court is not bound to hold that a doctor escapes liability for negligent treatment or diagnosis just because he followed a protocol or guideline.

The probative authority of guidelines and protocols was examined in the case of Early-v- Newham [1994] 5 Med LR 214.
Facts of the case:
A patient suffered a terrifying experience during induction of anaesthesia. Induction was unsuccessful and she woke up still paralysed by suxamethonium. The Anaesthetic SHO had followed the local protocol 'to maintain cricoid pressure, ventilate with oxygen, not persist with attempts at intubation, turn the patient on the side, call for help...... allow the patient to wake up'.

The claimant alleged that the guideline was faulty and flawed and her expert advised the court that no 'reasonably competent medical authority would have condoned this drill'. The judge found that the anaesthetic drill have been properly considered by the Anaesthetic department. The risks involved had been balanced, considering the risk of transient terror to be outweighed by the risk of hypoxia or aspiration. The department's protocol had therefore been reasonable and competent.

Departure from accepted practice: If a doctor deviates from the accepted practice (guideline/protocol) this is not in itself negligent but he must be able to justify his actions. The decision may well be justified by the particular circumstances of the patient, it being remembered that doctors have to treat the individual patient and not the 'standard patient'. A substantial departure from accepted practice, even taken consciously and in full knowledge of the potential risks, will place a heavy burden on the doctor to justify the decision. The doctor having taken a conscious decision to depart from the accepted practice, must exercise professional judgement about the balance of risks and benefits attached to a proposed treatment.

A deviation from ordinary professional practice is not necessarily evidence of negligence. Even a substantial deviation from normal practice may be warranted by the particular circumstances. Generally, the more serious the damage, the more difficult it will be for the doctor to justify his actions.

In *Clark-v- MacLennan* *[1983] 1ALL ER 416,* the judge held that the defendants had not justified their departure from standard practice and were thus liable.

Facts of the case:
The claimant developed stress incontinence after giving birth. The doctor operated within 4weeks of the birth. The operation and two subsequent repairs also failed. The accepted practice was that the operation should not have been performed until at least three months after the birth.

Pain J stated: ' where …there is but one orthodox course of treatment and the doctor chooses to depart from that, ….it is not enough to say as to his decision simply that it was based on his judgement. One has to inquire whether he took all the proper facts into account which he knows or should have known, and whether his departure from the orthodox course can be justified on the basis of these factors'.

Current Practice:

Electronic library has made access to medical information in other parts of the world available through electronic libraries and databases. It is therefore pertinent that the practice the courts are willing to endorse is defined. Whilst there is no case law to date on this point that is not to say that this cannot be referred to in a medical negligence claim. My submission on this is that the reference to accepted practice should be clinical practice in the U.K. Otherwise there will be varying standards of care and an onerous burden on the clinician to keep abreast with practices in other continents. Where an NHS Trust treat their patients in abroad, the accepted practice will be that prevailing in the state at the time despite being under the care of the NHS Trust.

SUMMARY

- Accepted practice must be current practice. A doctor cannot doggedly stick to outdated practice.

- The judicial emphasis placed on compliance with accepted practice means that a professional person is obliged to update their knowledge continually in order to ensure that new developments within the profession are incorporated into practice.

- This does not mean that every new technique must be adopted nor does it mean that every publication must be read – all he is required to do is to act responsibly and reasonably.

- Guidelines, protocols and Integrated Care Pathways are the usual evidence of what is accepted practice.

- The courts in deciding what is the standard of care place a heavy reliance on the expert witness – a body of opinion which is responsible and reasonable.

- The courts can reject a body of opinion if it does not withstand judicial scrutiny or demonstrate a logical basis for its opinion.

- A professional person 'should not lag behind other ordinary assiduous and intelligent members of the profession in knowledge of new advances, discoveries and developments in the field.' Eckersley- v- Binnie (1988) 18 Con LR1.

References
1. GMC – Duties of a doctor : Good Medical Practice (1995)
2. GMC - Serious Communicable Diseases (2004)

Statutes
1. Congenital Disabilities (Civil Liability) Act 1976
2. Consumer Protection Act 1987
3. The Sale of Goods & Supply of Service Act 1974
4. The Sale and Supply of Goods Act 1994

Caselaw
1. Barnett –v- Chelsea & Kensington Hospital Management Committee [1968] 1 All ER 1068
2. Bolam-v- Friern Barnet Health Management Committee [1957] 1 WLR 582
3. Bolitho-v- City and Hackney Health Authority [1993] 4MLR 381
4. Burton-v- Islington HA {1993] 4 MLR 8
5. Caparo-v-Dickman [1990] 1 All ER 568
6. Clark-v- MacLenna [1983] 1 All 416
7. Early-v-Newham [1994] 5 MLR 214
8. Elder-v- Greenwich & Deptford Hospital Management Committee
9. Herican-v- Ruan [1991] 3 All ER 65
10. Holgarth-v- Lancashire Mental Hospital Board [1937]
11. Holmes-v- Board of Hospital Trustees of the City of London (1997) 81 DLR
12. Hotson-v- East Berkshire Area HA [1987] 2 All ER 909
13. Hucks-v- Cole [1994] MLR 393, CA
14. Hunter-v- Harley (1995) SLT 213 Scotland
15. Lloyd Cheyham & Co Ltd-v- Littlejohn & Co Ltd (1985) 2PN 154
16. McKay-v- Essex AHA (1982) QB 1166
17. Maynard-v- West Midland Regional HA [1984] 1 WLR 634
18. Newell and Newell –v- Goldenberg (1995)

19. Payne –v- St Helier GP HMCC (1952
20. Pittman Estate -v- Bain (1994) 112 DLR 4th 257
21. Ravenscroft-v- Rederiaktiebolaget Transatlantic [1991] 3 All ER 73, 84-5
22. Reay-v- BNF; Hope-v- BNF Plc [1994] 1WLR 582
23. Roe-v- Min of Health [1954] 2QB 66,83
24. Walters –v- North Glamorgan NHS Trust [2002] EWH 321 QB
25. Wilsher –v- Essex HA [1987] QB, CA [1988]. AC 1074 HL

Chapter 3
INFORMED CONSENT

Introduction:

The first part of this chapter will deal with the general principle of the doctrine of informed consent and in the second part, the principles will be applied to Obstetrics practice.

The Ethical basis of Consent

The ethical principle that every person has a right to self determination and respect of their autonomy finds its expression through the notion of consent. Informed consent as it applies to medical practice affords protection to the patient and the right to decide what is to happen to him.

The right to self determination is summed in the classic statement of Justice Cardozo: 'Every human being of adult years and sound mind has a right to determine what shall be done with his own body; and a surgeon who performs an operation without his patient's consent commits an assault, for which he is liable in damages'.
(Schloendorff-v- Society of New York Hospital 211 NY 125(1914).

Regardless of the doctor's opinion, it is the patient who has the final say on whether to undergo the treatment. If a doctor were to proceed in the face of a decision to reject treatment, he would be liable for his unauthorised conduct. Liability can stem in the criminal law as assault or battery, or in tort as battery or negligence. This is expressed succinctly in the words of Wall J in *Re JT (Adult : Refusal of Medical Treatment [1998] 1*

FLR 48 'it is in general terms a criminal and tortuous assault to perform physical invasive treatment without a patient's consent'

The legal basis of Consent

The ethical notion of self determination is judicially expressed as the legal basis for consent. It is frequently stated by judges that the right of self determination is a governing form for both medical treatment and other forms of conduct where the individual's physical integrity is compromised. Both the criminal and civil law recognise that there is a broad symbolic importance in the theory that the individual's body is inviolate. Protection of patient autonomy and individual rights is the bedrock of the legal basis of informed consent. Three areas of law provide the legal framework for the doctrine of informed consent as follows:

- Human Rights

    In the current climate of rights it is not far fetched to find protection within the Human Rights Act 1998.The right to determine what can be done to oneself is found in the 'right to privacy' under article 8 (1) European Convention of Human Rights (ECHR).Treatment without consent or forced treatment against the wishes of a competent patient could also be in breach of article 3 'not to be subject to inhuman or degrading treatment'

- Criminal Law

Any unauthorised touching is technically an assault even if there is no evidence of damage to the patient. It may seem harsh to hold that a doctor is criminally liable when the only thing that he is 'guilty of is trying to help another human being. There is a judicial reluctance and antipathy to find doctors liable for battery hence the paucity of caselaw in which a doctor has been prosecuted for assault/battery on his patient on grounds that consent was not obtained. Caselaw from other jurisdictions recognises that the only place for battery actions in medicine would be where there is an element of fraud or misrepresentation to the patient in relation to the treatment.

- Civil Law

a. Battery: This is a form of trespass to the person which is committed by intentionally bringing about a harmful or offensive contact with another person's body. The action therefore serves the dual purpose of affording protection to the individual not only against bodily harm but also against any interference with his person which is offensive to a reasonable sense of honour and dignity. If the doctor exceeds the scope of the consent given, this will be actionable under a claim for battery. In *Hamilton -v- Birmingham RHB [1969] 2 BMJ 456* the defendant was found liable for performing a sterilisation without consent during a caesarean section. In *Devi-v- West Midlands AHA (1981) CA*, the patient consented to an operation to repair her ruptured uterus, which had been punctured during another procedure. The surgeon whilst in the abdomen, believed it was in her best interests to perform a sterilisation. The Court of Appeal held that the doctor was liable for battery. It is prudent for the doctor obtaining the consent to anticipate and discuss with the patient the scope of further/alternative procedures as may be found necessary during the course of the planned procedure. This is not a panacea to carry out unnecessary procedures. It must be necessary and in the patient's best interest.

b. Negligence

Most civil actions and complaints in the remit of consent arises from patients who having consented to treatment, allege that they have simply not been told enough about what was going to happen, particularly the risks involved in order to make an informed choice. This is a specific medical negligence action. The legal issue is whether a duty of disclosure exists and if so what is the standard.

<u>Duty of disclosure:</u> As a matter of fact and law the duty to inform arises from the patient/doctor relationship not only to acts but also omissions, in this case the failure to properly inform. If the patient is entitled to be informed, the doctor is under a duty to provide the information. The purpose of the duty of disclosure is to enable a competent patient to make an informed choice about their medical care and strengthen their

autonomy. This is explicitly stated by Lord Diplock :

'To decide what risks the existence of which a patient should be voluntarily warned and the terms in which such warning, if any should be given…..is as much an exercise of professional skill and judgement as any other part of the doctor's comprehensive duty of care.' *Sidaway –v- Board of Governors of the Bethlehem Royal Hospital and the Maudsley Hospital [1985] 1 AC871 pg 895*

In this case the House of Lords imposed a duty on doctors to disclose information about risks associated with proposed medical treatment thus establishing a common law duty of disclosure of risks. A competent patient must be told about the risks of the proposed medical procedure. The doctor must take into 'account all the relevant considerations, which include the ability of the patient to comprehend what he has to say and the state of the patient at the particular time both from physical point of view and the emotional point of view……' Lord Woolf MR in *Pearce –v- United Bristol Healthcare NHS Trust (1998) 48 BMLR (CA)*

Professional obligations and the law require doctors to take reasonable steps in an attempt to ensure that patients understand the risks they are being asked to take, so facilitating meaningful choices and the opportunity to give a properly informed choice.

Standard of disclosure

The standard of care levied in medical matters is determined by the Bolam test: 'a practice which is accepted as proper by a responsible body of skilled and experienced doctors'. In the realm of disclosure the professional standard – what a reasonable body would think it appropriate for the patient to know was contested in the case of *Sidaway* .

Facts of the case:
The plaintiff had an operation to relieve her recurrent neck and shoulder pain. The operation carried a risk of damage to a nerve root of 1-2%. There was also a substantially smaller risk to her spinal cord. She was informed of the risk to the nerve root but the surgeon did not refer to the risk of paralysis that might result from damage to her spinal cord. The operation was performed competently, but the risk to her spinal cord materialised and she was left severely disabled. The

plaintiff sued the surgeon for failing to inform of this risk.

The case set out succinctly as a matter of law what the standard of care is in the realm of disclosure of risks. Four key principles were established:

1. It is a basic concept that a competent adult has a right to choose what shall happen to his or her body.
2. The consent is the informed exercise of a choice, and that entails the opportunity to evaluate knowledgeably the options available and the risks attendant to each.
3. The doctor must therefore disclose all material risks; what risks are 'material' is determined by the prudent patient test. This test uses a template what the reasonable patient, in the plaintiff's position would attach significance to in coming to a decision on treatment advice given.
4. Informed consent is subject to an overriding therapeutic privilege: if the information concerning the risk is detrimental to the health of the patient, then it need not be disclosed.

Risk Disclosure in the consent process

In Sidaway, risks were quantified in various terms: (a) substantial (b) general, (c) special (d) material . What do all these terms mean in practical terms? Are these risks to be regarded in terms of percentages which will bring the final analysis to a mathematical one. Discussion of the size of the risk in isolation overlooks the fact that in risk prediction, it is not only the existence of the risk that is important but what is the consequence of the risk which is helpful for the patient in making an informed choice.

A procedure may have a high risk of a long term benign condition whereas another may run a low risk with permanent and disabling outcome. What is grave or adverse is relative and a matter for the patient to decide.

Lord Templeman in Sidaway explored the meanings of some of these risk concept.

- Substantial risk: 'a risk so obviously necessary to an informed choice on the part of the patient that no reasonably prudent medical man would fail to make it'

- General risk: Ordinarily would be known to the patient and no duty to disclose would arise. These will be one that attends to all medical procedures e.g. infection, bleeding, pain

- Special risks: Call for specific mention by the doctor. One that is inherent in the particular procedure either because of the nature of the procedure itself or because of some circumstances particular to that patient. It may be special in kind, magnitude or special to the patient.

- Material risk: These are concerned with what a reasonable patient would want to know. In the Canadian case of Reibl-v-Hughes (1980) 114 DLR (3d)(1)CanSC 10% risk of stroke was cited as material. A word of caution here, as to percentages which is only helpful as to the likelihood of the risk occurring but not determinative of a general or special risk.

A general or special risk may be relevant to materiality but not conclusive. Whether a risk is significant or material cannot simply be equated to percentage figures. A significant risk may not necessarily be one that would determine the patient's choice to consent, but one that a reasonable patient would consider relevant to rather than conclusive of the choice made.

Practice Points

The NHSLA has issued an alert on informed consent with the following recommendation: (NHSLA Risk Alert Issue 4, Nov 2004)

- Extreme care in the taking of consent is even more crucial than ever
- Careful and comprehensive warnings about all significant possible adverse outcomes must be given
- The information given must be carefully recorded in the notes
- The patient should be invited to sign the entry to confirm that he/she has been given the warning, has understood it and accepts the risk.
- It is equally important to make a full entry in the notes, preferably signed by the patient, if treatment is refused including the reason.

The process of informed consent.

For a consent to be valid it must be given voluntarily by an appropriately informed person, who has the capacity to consent for examination or treatment. All forms of consent therefore require the elements of competence, information and voluntariness.

- Competence

There is a presumption that an adult patient has the necessary mental capacity to consent or refuse consent to medical treatment. The onus will be upon those who seek to argue that the patient is indeed mentally incompetent to show this.

In general, to be considered competent an individual must be able to comprehend the nature of the particular conduct in question and to understand its quality and consequences. Competence is on a sliding scale- a person may be considered competent to consent for one procedure but not another. Neither is a person incompetent because of mental illness. There are two approaches in the determination of competence- capacity and the status approach.

- Capacity:

The capacity approach focuses on the individual's actual functioning in the decision making process. In applying this approach what is relevant is whether someone is in fact capable of making a particular decision as judged by the consistency between the person's choice and the individual's underlying values and by the extent to which the choice promotes the individual's well being as he or she sees it.

The legal test of capacity is set out in the case of Re C

(Adult: Refusal of Treatment)(1994)

Facts of the case:

C was 68years old with paranoid schizophrenia. He developed gangrene in the foot and the clinical team responsible for his care felt that an amputation was required to prevent the spread of the gangrene. C applied for and was granted an injunction preventing the amputation being carried out. This was despite the fact that there was an 85% chance that death would result, and the refusal would soon be irrevocable because C's mental state was deteriorating .The judge in allowing C's injunction against treatment considered the relevant question regarding capacity to be

'whether C's capacity is so reduced by his chronic mental illness that he does not sufficiently understand the nature, purpose and effects of the treatment.'

The court in granting C's injunction formulated a 3 stage test of capacity:
a. comprehending and retaining treatment information
b. believing it
c. weighing it in the balance to arrive at a choice.

The above three criteria are now the legal test of competence in English law. These requirements must be applied in conjunction with the Mental Health Act 1983 and the Mental Health Act code when treatment is related to a mental illness.

Any doctor can make an assessment of competence if the patient has 'their wits around them'. Where there is doubt a psychiatrist opinion should be sought.

In the determination of competence the Court of Appeal in *St George's Healthcare NHS Trust –v- S (1998) 3 All ER 673* laid down the following guidelines:

i. The authority should identify as soon as possible whether there is concern about a patient's competence to consent or refuse treatment.

ii. If the capacity of the patient is seriously in doubt, it should be assessed as a matter of priority. In many cases the patient's GP or other responsible doctor may be sufficiently qualified to make the necessary assessment, but in serious or complex cases involving difficult issues about future health and well being or even the life of the patient, the issue of capacity should be examined by an independent psychiatrist.

- Status

This approach sets a single and specific cut off point for the determination of competence, with a presumption that those deemed incompetent would be incapable in law of making some overall treatment decisions. Minors and patients with mental illness or unconscious would therefore be deemed incapable of making decisions about their treatment without regard to their actual capabilities. Whilst this is true for the unconscious patient, the other two groups may actually be able to make treatment choices. The fact that a patient belongs to a group of persons who are often unable to make general decisions for their own well being should alert the health carer to the probability of decisional incapacity but it is not conclusive of it. This is particularly demonstrated in older children who are able to make healthcare decisions for themselves. The leading case which established a principle in the way decisions by minors are determined is the case of

Gillick-v- West Norfolk and Wisbech AHA [1986] AC 112, [1985] 3 All ER 402

Facts of the case:

The Department of Health and Social Security issued guidance to local Health Authorities concerning family planning services for young persons under the age of 16 years. The advice emphasised the importance of involving the parents but added that in exceptional circumstances the doctor could prescribe contraceptive without informing the parents. Mrs Gillick sought a judicial review that the guidance was unlawful.

The House of Lords held that a child under the age of 16 years could, in law, have the capacity to consent and that ability to understand was the key to competence.

Lord Fraser laid down five requirements that should be satisfied before the doctor concludes that he may proceed without the parent's consent.

1. That the girl will understand the advice

INFORMED CONSENT

2. That he cannot persuade her to inform her parents or to allow him to inform the parents that she is seeking contraceptive advice.
3. That she is very likely to begin or continue having sexual intercourse with or without contraceptive treatment
4. That unless she receives contraceptive advice or treatment her physical or mental health or both are likely to suffer;
5. That her best interest require him to give her contraceptive advice, treatment or both without parental consent.

The 'Fraser' guideline ('*Gillick* competence) applies to persons under 16 years who has a consistent pattern of development. The Gillick decision does not remove the right of consent from the parent. Therefore parental consent can override a refusal of consent made by a competent minor. The converse of course is that the person with parental responsibility cannot override the consent of the competent minor.

- Information

    The duty of the doctor in the realm of disclosure of information is two-fold. The first and most fundamental of this legal duty is to provide the patient with information of the broad nature and purpose of the procedure. The scope of that duty has already been explored comprehensively in the earlier part of this chapter. To that I will add that the duty to inform is a continuing one and information must be disclosed prior to, during and after the procedure. The doctor must disclose all the material risks and alternative forms of treatment. Similarly if a medical accident occurs in the course of treatment, the patient or their relatives if appropriate must be informed.

    The second ambit of that legal duty is that the doctor should ensure at least a degree of understanding on the part of the patient. Unless the patient understands the information they are given, they will be no better off and disclosure would have been a mock exercise. The patient must be able to understand the information which is material to the discussion especially as to the likely consequences of having or not having the treatment in question.

    The medical profession appears increasingly to acknowledge that it is bound to go beyond merely providing information by taking steps to ensure that what is said is comprehended. The standard consent forms currently in use in NHS hospitals, for example, require that the doctor ' confirm that I have explained the operation…in terms which, in my judgement are suited to the understanding of the patient'.

The Royal College of Surgeons in its guidance - The surgeons duty of care- Guidance for surgeons on ethical and legal issues, 1998, at 6 declares that 'surgeons should satisfy themselves that the choices of patients are the result of understanding and deliberation about information provided concerning diagnosis and treatment'.

The GMC in its guidance, Seeking Patient's Consent : the ethical considerations 1999, advice doctors 'that patients need to understand what they are being told and the doctor must consider how well patients have appreciated the implication of what is proposed'.(para 27)

The information process should use simple understandable words and include if appropriate discussion about any patient related factors e.g occupation, surgical history which could affect the risks and the desirability of a particular outcome.

- Voluntariness

    A valid consent should be free from duress, undue influence and misrepresentation.

    When obtaining consent it is often preferable especially with elective procedure to allow the patient a 'cooling off' period after full discussion of the planned procedure and obtain written consent later. This may be difficult for administrative reasons and a procedure often adapted by many hospitals is a pre-assessment clinic a few weeks before the procedure to allow any further enquiries and reaffirm the consent already given.

PARTICULAR PROBLEMS

In this section, some particular problems that may arise in clinical practice will be explored. These are namely treatment of the incompetent minor, the incompetent adult, in an emergency situation and refusal of treatment.

- Emergency Treatment

    This refers especially to the unconscious patient, the incompetent adult or minor. In an emergency the need for care is obvious and in the words of Sir Thomas Bingham

    'I have in mind the acute emergency when a decision has to be taken within minutes or at most hours as to whether treatment should be given or not, whether one form of treatment should be given or another or as to whether treatment should be withheld'. *(Frenchay Healthcare NHS Trust -v- S [1994]2 All 403 pg409).*

    As these group of persons cannot give consent it is therefore not required in an emergency. As such the healthcarer must normally 'act in the best interests of the patient'. This means that the treatment is limited to that which is necessary to save life or to ensure improvement or prevent deterioration in physical and mental health.

    There are three necessary requirements for the application of the doctrine of necessity:

    i. The act is needed to avoid inevitable and irreparable evil

    ii. No more should be done than is reasonably necessary for the purpose to be achieved;

    iii. The evil inflicted must not be disproportionate to the evil avoided.

    In an unconscious patient, if the unconsciousness is likely to last for some time but the treatment is immediately necessary then treatment can be administered in the patient's best interest. If the treatment is not immediately needed then much will depend on when the patient is likely to regain consciousness and what is immediately necessary. If the unconsciousness will only last for a short time then only emergency treatment that will improve the patient's condition should be given and all other elective treatment deferred until the patient regains consciousness. Where the patient has a valid advance directive, necessity cannot override the competently made advance directive.

    In an emergency situation the legal right of consent does not pass to a relative. Whilst their views and wishes should be listened to and it is best practice to consult with them to avoid tension arising, they cannot determine, veto or give consent in the circumstance. The real practice difficulty is who in the medical team makes the decision and decides what and how the patient's best interests are to be determined.

- The Incompetent Adult

    This discussion refers to therapeutic treatment for the incompetent adult such as those with dementia, persistent vegetative state and learning disability. Treatment of a mentally incompetent patient for a mental illness under the Mental Health Act 1983 is excluded in this discussion which is outside the scope of this book. As the patients in the clinical condition described above are unable to give consent, the common law allows the health carer to do what is in the patient's best interest. Spouses and relatives have no legal power to consent or refuse treatment on behalf of incompetent adults.

    The views of the relatives are to be considered to assist the health carer in determining the patient's best interests. This encompasses medical, emotional and all the other welfare issues, whether the patient had a preference on what treatment should be administered and whether treatment should continue in a given situation. In determining what is in the best interests of the patient, section 4 of the Mental Capacity Act 2005 provides a statutory framework for decision making:

    1. The ascertainable past and present wishes of the person and the factors the person would consider if able to do so;
    2. The need to permit and encourage the person to participate in any decision affecting him;
    3. The views of other people whom it is appropriate and practical to consult;
    4. Whether the purpose can be as effectively achieved in a manner less restrictive of the person's freedom of action;
    5. Whether there is a reasonably foreseeable future;
    6. The need to be satisfied that the wishes of the person without capacity were not the result of undue influence.

    The health care makes the ultimate decision in the patient's 'best interest'.

There is an ignorance amongst the medical profession that the next of kin should be asked to consent on behalf of the incompetent adult. In English law, a proxy cannot make give consent on behalf of an adult. The law in this area is likely to change with the Mental Capacity Act 2005, which allows the appointment of a welfare attorney who will be able to make decisions on behalf of the incompetent adult. Where non therapeutic treatment is contemplated in the best interests of the patient e.g adult female sterilisation the prior permission of the court should be sought.

- The Incompetent Minor

  The person with parental responsibility is permitted to give consent on behalf of the child. The legal and ethical considerations here is the basis and extent to which that consent applies. The proxy consenting is not at liberty to make whatever decision he or she pleases. The breadth of the power to consent is underpinned by the best interests of the child. The concept of best interests is given statutory recognition in s1(1) of the Children Act 1989 in the welfare principle. Best interests or welfare of the child is issue specific and fact based. Various pieces of legislation also give the power of consent to others who may need it from time to time. For example :

  - A person who does not have parental responsibility for a particular child, but has care of the child e.g. teachers and childminders. Such a person 'may do what is reasonable in all the circumstances of the case for the purpose of safeguarding and promoting the child's welfare especially in an emergency

  - The wardship jurisdiction of the Crown Court has the power of consent where a minor is concerned to protect the child from the actions or motivations of others. In exercising that jurisdictional power, the child is made a ward of the court. The court is therefore obliged to make decisions in the best interests of the child which overrides the rights of the parents.

  - The local authority may apply to the court in a care proceedings to exercise parental responsibility over the child and thereby make proxy decisions on behalf of the child.

Tensions can arise between the parents and the health care team necessitating a resort to the courts for a declaration. This may arise where the parents insists on treatments which are futile(life prolonging treatments, CPR) or non therapeutic treatments e.g. sterilisation . Tactful consultation and mediation with all the parties should resolve the tension but if this fails the leave of the court should be sought. The courts would not exercise its inherent jurisdiction over minors by ordering a medical practitioner to treat the minor in a manner contrary to the practitioners clinical judgement. To do so would require the practitioner to act contrary to the fundamental duty which he owed to his patient, which is to treat the patient in accordance with his own best clinical judgement.

The courts are therefore reluctant to dictate treatment as the courts must take decisions that are in the child's best interests. In R-v-Portsmouth Hospitals NHS Trust ex p Carol Glass (1999) the Court of Appeal laid out a number of principles that the court should take into account when intervening on decisions whether or not to treat a child:

a. The sanctity of life

b. The non interference by the courts in areas of clinical judgement in the treatment of patients......where this can be avoided.

c. The refusal of the courts to dictate appropriate treatment to a medical practitioner subject to the power which the courts always have to take decisions in relation to the child's best interests. In doing so, the court takes fully into account the attitude of medical practitioners.

d. That treatment without consent save in an emergency is trespass to the person

e. That the courts will interfere to protect the interests of a minor or a person under a disability.

- Refusal of Treatment

    The right of self determination encompasses the right to refuse medical treatment. A competent adult is generally entitled to refuse a specific treatment or all treatment, or to select an alternative form of treatment, even if the decision may entail risks as serious as death and may appear mistaken in the eyes of the medical profession or others. When a patient refuses treatment, in principle the doctor's duty may extend to advising the patient of the consequences of the decision. The California Supreme Court found that the failure to advice a female patient of the consequences of refusing a smear test could constitute a breach of duty by the doctor, when she subsequently died from cervical cancer.

The right to refuse treatment was endorsed by Lord Goff : '.. it is established that the principle of self determination requires that respect must be given to the wishes of the patient, so that, if an adult patient of sound mind refuses, however unreasonably, to consent to treatment or care by which his life would or might be prolonged, the doctors responsible for his care must give effect to his wishes, even though they do not consider it to be in his best interests to do so. To this extent, the principle of the sanctity of life must yield to the principle of self determination'. (*Airedale NHS Trust- v- Bland [1993] AC 789,HL*)

Patients refusing treatment will often have the issue of capacity raised especially if the refusal is unfathomable or absurd. This was exactly the issue raised in the case of *Re T (Adult Refusal of Medical Treatment) [1992] 3 WLR 782, CA*

Facts of the case:

T was a pregnant woman Jehovah's witness who refused life saving blood transfusion. She required a caesarean section to which she refused to give consent and post operatively required a blood transfusion. The Court of Appeal held that her decision to refuse surgery and blood transfusion was invalid because it was based solely upon the persuasion of her mother who was a Jehovah's witness.

An irrational decision may call into question the competence of the patient but it is not conclusive of incompetence.

'A competent person who has the capacity to decide may, for rational or irrational reasons or for no reason at all, choose not to have medical intervention though the consequences may be death or serious handicap of the child she bears or her own death' Butler-Sloss LJ in *Re MB (Medical Treatment)(1997)*.

Patients autonomy demands that the patient's choice should be respected even if that decision is outrageous in its defiance of logic or accepted moral standards that no sensible person could have arrived at that decision. To a large extent a patient's belief system, culture and race will influence their decision and this should be respected rather than raising the issue of competence on the actual decision provided the patient has the capacity to make the decision.

Incompetent patients have no legal right to refuse consent but a distinction must be made between patients with psychiatric illness and still competent to refuse treatment and those who lack capacity. If treatment is in the best interests of the incompetent patient, then treatment must be given despite the refusal. This will also apply to patients above the age of 16years but under 18years old who have a statutory right to consent under s8 of the Family Law Reform Act 1969.

In ReW (A Minor) (Medical Treatment) [1992] 3 WLR 758, CA Lord Donaldson stated that ' No minor of whatever age has power by refusing consent to treatment to override a consent to treatment by someone who has parental responsibility for the minor and a consent by the court. Nevertheless such a refusal is a very important consideration in making clinical judgement and for parents and the courts in deciding whether themselves to give consent. Its importance increases with the age and maturity of the minor.

INFORMED CONSENT

SUMMARY

- The informed consent of the patient is a prerequisite for any medical intervention.
- A valid consent can only be given by an appropriately informed person who has the capacity to consent and voluntarily.
- Capacity is the ability to understand the information relevant to the decision, retain that information, use or weigh that information as part of the process of making decisions and communicate that decision.
- The patient has the right to refuse or discontinue a medical treatment. The implication of doing so must be carefully explained to the patient.
- The law requires not only that the doctor provide information to the patient prior to or as part of the medical treatment, but also that the doctor must take reasonable steps to ensure that the information is adequate in scope, content and presentation, to convey the risks of, alternatives to the treatment; is intelligible to the particular patient having regard to all the circumstances of the patient and is understood by the patient.
- When a patient is unable to express his or her will and a medical intervention is urgently required the consent of the patient may be presumed unless it is obvious from a previously declared expression of will that consent would be refused in the situation.
- A doctor can proceed with treatment in the absence of a legal representative or proxy decision maker if the intervention is too urgent to wait as an act of necessity in the best interests of the patient.
- If the proxy refuses consent and the physician is of the opinion that the intervention is in the interests of the patient, an independent committee (e.g. ethics committee) or as a last resort a court should review the decision.
- A lack of capacity cannot be established merely by reference to a person's age, appearance or a condition of his or an aspect of his behaviour, which might lead others to make unjustified assumptions about his capacity.

References:
1. NHS LA, 'NHSLA Risk Alert' Issue 4 Nov 2004
2. General Medical Council : Seeking Patient's Consent The Ethical considerations
3. General Medical Council: Good Medical Practice (2001)
4. The Senate of Surgery of Gt Britain & Ireland, The Surgeons duty of care. Guidance for surgeons on ethical and legal issues.1998
5. RCOG: Clinical Governance Advice No 6 Oct 2004- Obtaining valid consent
6. Medical Ethics Today. BMJ Books 2004

Case Law:
1. Airedale NHS trust –v- Bland [1993] AC 789,HL
2. Devi-v- West Midlands AHA (1981) AC 112
3. Frenchay Healthcare NHS trust-v- S [1994] 2All 403
4. Gillick-v- West Norfolk and Wisbech AHA [1986] AC 112, HL
5. Hamilton-v- Birmingham RHB [1969] 2 bmj 456
6. Pearce-v- United Bristol Healthcare NHS Trust (1999) 48 BMLR 118, CA
7. Re C (Adult : Refusal of Treatment)[1994] 1 WLR 290
8. Re JT (Adult: Refusal of Medical Treatment [1998] 1FLR 48
9. Re J (A minor) (Wardship: Medical Treatment) [1992] 4 All ER 614, CA
10. Re MB (Medical Treatment) [1997] 2 FLR 426, CA
11. Re T (Adult Refusal of Medical Treatment)[1992] 3 WLR 782, CA
12. Re W (A minor) (Medical Treatment) [1992] 3 WLR 758, CA
13. R-v- Portsmouth Hospitals NHS Trust exp Carol Glass [1999] Lloyd's LR Med 367, CA
14. Reibl-v- Hughes (1980) 114 DLR CanSC
15. Schloendorff-v- Society of New York Hospital 211 NY 125(1914)
16. Sidaway-v- Board of Governors of the Royal Bethlehem Royal Hospital and Maudsley Hospital [1985] 1AC 871, HL
17. St Georges Healthcare NHS Trust-v- S [1998] 3All ER 673,CA

Chapter 4
CONSENT IN OBSTETRICS

INTRODUCTION

It is the patient's right to autonomy that lies at the heart of the principle of consent. The patient has the right to choose whether or not to undergo a specific treatment being recommended by her doctor. The patient has to be provided with all the relevant information and knowledge about the procedure at hand before making any decision and the duty falls on the doctor to provide this information. A conflict may arise when the patient's choice is contrary to accepted medical practice.

WHAT IS CONSENT?

In law, valid consent from the patient prevents an operation or any other invasive treatment performed from being an assault (or trespass to the person). Valid consent is obtained when consent is voluntarily given by a person who is appropriately informed of the risks, benefits and alternatives of the procedure at hand, provided the person being consented has the requisite legal capacity to give it. In considering a patient's capacity the court can apply the 3 stage test set out in Re C (1994) which provides that the patient must be able to:-

1. Comprehend and retain relevant information;

2. Believe it; and
3. Weigh it in the balance so as to arrive at a choice.

Any decision to refuse treatment by a patient who has capacity must be respected regardless of whether it is neither sensible, rational nor well considered. There are 2 forms of consent; express (written) or implied. The validity of consent does not depend on the form in which it is given. Written consent is required for surgery or there can be implicit consent for other less invasive forms of treatment. Both forms of consent require the elements discussed above, i.e. understanding of the nature of the treatment (competence), sufficient information to reach a decision as to whether to refuse or consent to the treatment (knowledge) and finally willingness to undergo the treatment (voluntary).

Where there is a failure to provide adequate information about a proposed procedure the physician may be considered to have breached his/her duty of care to the patient and therefore have acted negligently.

If the patient does not give valid consent to the procedure a claim may be brought for assault/trespass to the person.

OBTAINING CONSENT

Consent is based on full and open communication between the doctor and his/her patient. All discussions leading to consent should as a matter of good practice involve an exchange of information and consideration of the patient's wishes. The patient should be given the opportunity to question the doctor and obtain all the information that she requires in order to make an informed decision as to whether to consent or not. The patient needs to understand the nature and purpose of the procedure. Any failure by a doctor to provide the patient with this broad understanding of the procedure may result in allegations of negligence. It was decided by the House of Lords in the leading case of Sidaway –v– Board of Governors of Bethlem Royal Hospital (1985) that the legal test to be applied when considering whether a doctor was negligent in relation to the provision of advice about treatment was the same as that set in the case of Bolam; a doctor would not be held to have acted negligently in the consent process if he acted in accordance with a reasonable body of medical opinion. A doctor owes a duty of care to a patient he/she chooses to treat and has a duty to inform a patient of any risks inherent in a procedure. Some risks, however, might be thought to be so rare that under Sidaway a doctor who failed to mention these would not be held to have acted negligently provided he/she could establish that his/her practice was supported by others offering the same procedure (but see later).

PATIENT'S RIGHT TO CHOOSE

The patient has no legal right to insist on her choice of treatment where that treatment is contrary to accepted medical practice. This can be seen most obviously in the context of caesarean sections. The number of women electing for caesarean sections is on the increase. Where the accepted practice is vaginal delivery should elective caesareans be performed? In a survey of female Obstetricians in London, 31% were found to choose delivery by caesarean section for themselves. However a woman doesn't have a legal right to insist on treatment which is contrary to accepted practice. An application for a court order compelling an Obstetrician to perform a caesarean section would fail if there was no clinical justification for it. The main reason given for not performing elective caesareans is maternal complications. However, this mode of delivery is now considered to be safe. There is also now evidence of instrumental delivery being associated with pelvic floor damage and incontinence. The New Zealand study of Wilson et al looked at the prevalence of urinary continence 3 months after delivery. When the data was analysed by method of delivery only 5.2% of the cohort who had delivered a first child by caesarean section had some evidence of urinary incontinence, compared to 24.5% of women who had their first delivery vaginally. As well as urinary incontinence, disruption of the anal sphincter is now also recognised as a complication of vaginal delivery. In the study of Sutton et al, 35% of the cohort undergoing a first vaginal delivery sustained damage to the internal and external anal sphincter. In a cohort of women undergoing first delivery by caesarean section, not a single woman developed a new anal sphincter defect.

Are women warned of the risks of sphincter defects? Are they warned of the risks of urinary stress incontinence especially after a number of vaginal deliveries? It may be worth far more to the individual to avoid these complications than to go through the process of a 'natural' vaginal delivery. There are associated risks with caesarean section but why do they remain clinically unjustifiable? Should the choice not be up to the woman who has to undergo the procedure as long as she is fully informed of all of the risks?

As a broad statement of law a foetus has no legal personality and rights. A woman can thus decline to undergo a caesarean section, contrary to medical advice, regardless of the potential consequences. In St Georges Healthcare Trust v. S (1998), a mother suffering from pre-eclampsia refused delivery by caesarean section despite being told of the risk to her and her child from a natural birth. The Court of Appeal found that even when his or her own life depended on receiving medical treatment, an adult of sound mind was entitled to refuse. The appellant's right to choose was not diminished because the decision to exercise it may appear "morally repugnant".

For the future, the advent of the Human Rights Act (HRA) 1998 has brought about the possibility of developing further legal rights. Article 2 of the European Convention of Human Rights imposes the positive duty to protect the right to life, although in Paton the European Commission of Human Rights ruled that Article 2 cannot apply to a foetus. The European Court of Human Rights is not bound by previous decisions and takes account of changing social attitudes. If a declaration was sought from the European Court where a woman refused a caesarean section, the Court would need to weigh in the balance the rights of the foetus against those of the mother under Article 2, under Article 3 which provides the right not to be subjected to inhuman or degrading behaviour and Article 8 which guarantees the right to private and family life.

In many commonly offered obstetric procedures, there are possible adverse consequences e.g. ARM, administration of syntocinon, the use of foetal scalp electrodes, the use of forceps and episiotomy. Written consent is not required, but a woman should be fully involved in the decision to undergo them. The consent process in episiotomy requires particular care. Since a woman's capacity to give informed consent during labour may be impaired by pain, stress and narcotics, information about the procedure should be provided well before labour has set in, thus allowing the woman the opportunity to ask any questions and obtain any information that she requires. If she has been fully informed and has given clear instructions, an episiotomy shouldn't present any consent problems in the delivery room in the event of an emergency. Where the woman has communicated her resolve not to undergo an episiotomy, and the obstetrician feels unable to exclude it becoming a medical necessity, the offer of caesarean section ought to be made. If her decision is ignored, there is lack of consent and the woman would have a claim for trespass.

There is no good reason why observance of this right (the woman's right to elect which of the foreseeable procedures she is willing to undergo) should not form part of standard obstetric practice and a legal remedy be available for a breach of it.

DEVELOPMENTS IN THE LAW OF CONSENT

The court's desire to preserve patients' autonomy has led to the majority decision of the Hose of Lords in the case of Chester v Afshar [2004]. It is still a matter of some uncertainty how this case will affect clinical negligence claims in the future. In that case Mrs Chester was advised by Mr Afshar, a spinal surgeon of considerable repute, to undergo back surgery. Despite his denial, it was found as a fact by the trial judge that Mr Afshar had failed to warn her of a 1-2% inherent risk that the operation might lead to cauda equina syndrome. This risk materialised without, as the judge found, any negligence on the part of Mr Afshar in his performance of the operation. The risk of cauda equina syndrome was a random risk inherent in the procedure being undertaken, irrespective of the skill of the surgeon performing it. There was nothing that the surgeon could have done to lower the risk.

On settled legal principles of causation, Mrs Chester was required to say that if she had been properly advised she would not have agreed to undergo the procedure recommended for her, and therefore would not have been exposed to the risk. In fact Mrs Chester could not say whether she would have chosen to undergo the procedure at some stage. However she did show to the judge's satisfaction that she would not have agreed to undergo the procedure which she did undergo because she would have sought a second opinion which would have taken time to obtain. Thus, it was argued, she would not have been under Mr Afshar's knife when the random risk occurred. But was that enough to provide her with a remedy?

The decision in the case involved a departure from acknowledged causation principles. A failure to advise was in itself a negligent act which a majority of their Lordships felt merited a remedy. Thus they abandoned traditional principles of legal causation on the policy grounds that the doctor's duty to warn of the risks of surgery would be a "hollow one", if Mrs Chester's honest uncertainty rendered her remedy-less.

Can the result in this case be elevated to provide a general remedy against the doctor who fails in his duty to inform adequately of risks or is it to be confined to its own facts? Is any failure to warn of a potential risk which then materialises through no fault of the practitioner themselves going to lead to a finding of negligence?

It might be considered that judges could be sceptical of the patient who claims to be in the same state of honest uncertainty as Mrs Chester was, just as they have been sceptical in the past where a claimant has asserted she would have declined a recommended operation because of some small but significant risk of complication.

The decision may have an impact where consent is obtained by one doctor, the patient's doctor of choice, but the procedure is in fact carried out by another doctor and an inherent risk materialises through no fault of the doctor. The Claimant might be able to argue that if they had been aware that her doctor of choice was not carrying out the operation she wouldn't have agreed to the surgery at that time.

CONCLUSION

At this stage it remains difficult to forecast the long term effect of the House of Lords decision in Chester. There are already signs that other members of the House of Lords will seek to limit the effect of the decision. In Gregg v Scott [2005]. Baroness Hale stated that the result does not alter 'the principles applicable to the great majority of personal injury cases'. In Moy v Pettman-Smith & Or, Lord Carswell indicated that the case in no way alters the requirement that patients must prove that they would, if properly warned, have declined to undergo the treatment in order to succeed in these claims.

The principle will thus be limited to the exceptional case where the patient is able to establish that she would not have undergone the actual operation if she had been given an adequate warning, but may have had it at a later date. The first limb of that proof has always been the hardest to establish and remains a requirement in law.

The basis of Lord Steyn's reasoning in Chester (he was one of the majority) appears to have been the failure to ensure that the patient had given her 'informed consent to the surgery in the full legal sense'. This has suggested to some commentators that the doctrine of 'informed consent' prevalent in the United States and parts of the Commonwealth is perhaps about to make itself felt in English law post HRA 1988 in preference to the approach in Sidaway outlined previously. The case of Pearce ~v~ United Bristol Healthcare NHS Trust (1999) refers to the patient's right to be warned of any "significant" risk. This case acknowledged the right to know on the part of patients.

The decision in Chester seems to illustrate the policy and corrective justice consideration that is pulling powerfully in favour of patients' rights to know.

References
1. Re C (Adult: Refusal of Medical Treatment) [1994] 1 ALL ER 819
2. Sidaway -v- Stopboard of Governors of Bethlem Royal Hospital [1985] AC 871
3. Bolam v Friern Hospital Management Committee [1957] 1 WLR 582
4. Department of Health. Changing Childbirth: Report of the Expert Maternity Group London: HMSO; 1993.
5. Wilson P D, Herbison RM, Herbison GP. Obstetric practice and the prevalence of urinary incontinence three months after delivery. Br J Obstet Gaynaecol 1996; 103:154-61.
6. Sutton AH, Kamm M, Hudson CN, Thomas JM, Bartram CI. Sphincter disruption during vaginal deliveries. N Engl J Med 1993; 329: 1905-11.
7. Paterson-Brown S. Should doctors perform an elective caesarean section on request? Yes, as long as the woman is fully informed. BMJ 1998;317:462-5.
8. Re MB [1997] 2 FLR 426 (CA)
9. St Georges Healthcare Trust v. S [1998] 3 ALL ER 673
10. Paton -v- United Kingdon [1980] 3 EHRR 408
11. Royal College of Obstetricians and Gynaecologists, Clinical Governance Advice, Obtaining Valid Consent, October 2004.
12. Chester v Afshar [2004] UKHL 41
13. Gregg v Scott [2005] UKHL 2
14. Moy v Pettman-Smith & Or [2005] UKHL 7
15. Pearce v United Bristol Healthcare NHS Trust [1998] BMLR 118/ [1999] PIQR P53

Chapter 5
CONFIDENTIALITY

In this chapter, it is proposed to explore the ethical and legal basis of confidentiality and clarify the doctors duty of care vis-à-vis disclosure to meet obligations in relation to confidentiality. Throughout this chapter reference will be made to the practice guidance issued by the GMC in the booklet 'Confidentiality : Protecting and Providing Information' (2004). The GMC guidance reflects good practice which would undoubtedly be supported by a court as practice 'accepted as proper by a responsible body of medical men'.

Confidence is the concept of trust not to disclose confidential information. The practical necessity of maintaining medical confidence is a fundamental part of clinical practice. The general rule is that information received in confidence for one purpose may not be used for another purpose or passed to anyone without the consent of the person who gave the confidential information. Confidential information includes all information relating to the employers' business, its patients and employees.

The Obligation of Confidence

The duty of confidence in the doctor-patient relationship lends support from the following areas

A. Ethics- The recognition of autonomy and control over information about oneself is one basis for the obligation of confidence. A utilitarian approach examines the interests that the obligation protects and the consequences of its violation i.e the balance of good and harm. Confidentiality protects from distress and facilitates trust in the health professional to whom he or she confides. This has a benefit that encourages and makes it more likely that the patient with embarrassing illnesses will seek help.

B. Trust & Confidence - The doctor –patient relationship is a fiduciary relationship and hence the confidant is under a duty of good faith to the confider. The information that ensues from such a relationship is imparted in circumstances importing obligations of confidence. In Fraser-v- Evans [1969] 1QB 349, CA Lord Denning MR stated: 'the jurisdiction for [confidentiality] is based not so much on property or on contract as on the duty to be of good faith. No person is permitted to divulge to the world information which he has received in confidence unless he has just cause or excuse for doing so'.

C. Professional Obligation - Patients have a right to expect that information about them will be held in confidence by their doctors. Confidentiality is central to trust between doctors and their patients. Without assurances about confidentiality, patients may be reluctant to give doctors the information they need in order to provide good care. This professional obligation is exemplified as follows:

- The Hippocratic Oath

'Whatsoever things I see or hear concerning the life of men, in my attendance on the sick or even apart therefrom, which ought not to be noised abroad, I will keep silence thereon, counting such things as sacred secrets'

- Declaration of Geneva

'I will respect the secrets which are confided in me, even if the patient has died'.

- General Medical Council

If you are asked to provide information about patients you should:
- seek patients consent to disclosure of information wherever possible , whether or not that patients can be identified from the

disclosure.
- anonymise data where unidentifiable data will serve the purpose
- keep disclosures to the minimum necessary
- you must always be prepared to justify your decisions in accordance with this guidance.

(GMC: Confidentiality- Protecting and Providing Information para 1 (2004))

- Legal

The legal duty of confidentiality is derived from (a) statutes and (b) the common law . The legal duty is identical to the ethical counterpart in its recognition of individual autonomy and the confiders' control of information about self.

Statute

I. Human Rights Act 1998

Confidentiality is a human right protected by the European Convention on Human Rights which is incorporated now into English law as the Human Rights Act 1998.

Article 8 provides for the right to respect for an individuals private and family life. This creates a right to privacy which is wider than the duty of confidentiality. The ECHR unequivocal view that confidential patient information is in principle protected from disclosure by art 8(1) is illustrated in the case *MS-v-Sweden (1997) 45 BMLR 133 (ECHR)*

Facts of the case :

MS made a claim for compensation under the Industrial Injury Insurance Act from the Social Insurance Office (SIO). During the proceedings, MS discovered that the SIO had requested and received, from the woman's clinic details from her medical records containing information that she had requested an abortion. MS had not been consulted about the disclosure. Her claim for compensation was rejected. In September 1992, MS lodged a complaint with the ECHR 'complaining that the submission of her medical records to the SIO constituted a violation of her right to respect for private and family life as guaranteed by art 8 of the ECHR 1950. The court observed that under the relevant Swedish law, the applicants' medical records at the clinic were governed by confidentiality, stressing that information of a private and sensitive nature had been disclosed without her consent to a certain number of people at the office. The measure constituted an interference with the applicant's right to respect for private life guaranteed by art 8 (1).

This case highlights potential unassuming breaches of confidence that can occur when one hospital department requests patient's medical records which had been collected and stored for medical treatment and its subsequent communication is to serve a different purpose. Clinicians must therefore guard against this and preferably seek legal advice or patient consent on requests for patients records for purposes outside medical treatment.

II. Data Protection Act 1998

Data protection law exists to strike a balance between the rights of individuals to privacy and ability of organisations to use data for legitimate business purposes.

The Data Protection Act (DPA) 1998 imposes obligations upon every person who holds and processes personal data on behalf of every data collected. The Act provides protection related to recorded data and not verbal confidences. The Act seeks to empower individuals and strengthen their rights about what is done to their personal and sensitive personal information. Within the Act, medical information is 'sensitive personal information'. Therefore the processing of such information is safeguarded by the conditions set out in schedule 3 of the Act:

- the patient must give explicit consent to the processing ;
- it must be necessary to protect patients 'vital interests' and they are unable to consent for themselves ;
- the processing is necessary for medical purposes and is undertaken by a health professional which includes preventive medicine, medical diagnosis, medical research, the provision of care and treatment and the management of healthcare services.

CONFIDENTIALITY

The underlying principles of the DPA 1998 are as follows: (sch 1,para 1-8)

Data shall be processed fairly and lawfully

1. A key component of the 'fair and lawful obligation is the need to inform the patients of the purposes to which information about them may be put. This means that patients should be informed of not only routine uses of their information, but also purposes such as clinical and administrative audits. This is an onerous duty that can be discharged by informing patients by way of leaflets enclosed with appointment letters and notices in waiting reception and consulting rooms.

2. Processed for limited purposes
   - Only use personal information for the purpose(s) for which it was obtained;
   - Only share information outside team or service if you are certain it is appropriate and necessary to do so.

3. Adequate, relevant and not excessive
   - Only collect and keep information you require.

4. Accurate and kept up to date.
   - Check information whenever possible to ensure accuracy.

5. Not kept for longer than is necessary.

6. Processed in line with individual rights.
   - Patients must be informed about what is being done with their information and how they can access their records.

7. Secure
   - All staff must know their responsibilities and patient information is only let to staff who need to know. Follow the employer's information security policy and code of practice for confidentiality.

8. Do not transfer to countries without adequate protection
   - If sending personal information outside the EEC, ensure consent is obtained and it is adequately protected.

The Rights of Data subjects under the Act

- Rights of access to records
- Right to prevent processing likely to cause damage or distress
- Right to prevent processing for purposes of direct marketing
- Rights in relation to automated decision making
- Right to compensation (where information is found to be inaccurate and or damaging and distressing)
- Right to apply to the Court for rectification, blocking, erasure and destruction
- Right to apply to the office of the information commissioner for assessment

III. NHS (Venereal Diseases) Regulations 1974(SI 1974, No29) NHS Trusts (Venereal Diseases) Directions 1991

These secondary legislation prohibit the disclosure of identifying information about a patient examined or treated for a sexually transmitted disease, other than to a medical practitioner, or to an individual under the direction of a medical practitioner in connection with and for the purpose of either the treatment of the patient and/or the prevention of the spread of the disease.

IV. S33 Human Fertilisation & Embryology Act 1990 as amended by the Human Fertilisation & Embryology (Disclosure of Information) Act 1992 :

Governs the circumstances in which information about patients may be disclosed by licensed centres.

V. Abortion Regulations 1991 (SI 1991 No 499)

Paragraph 5 requires that information supplied in an abortion notification has statutory restriction on disclosure of such information.

- Health Act 1999 ss23 & 24

This provides for statutory protection of information obtained by the Audit Commission in the carrying out of its functions which includes the collection and analysis of data which may comprise patient confidential information.

- Health Service Commissioners Act 1993 s15

This provides protection and restriction on disclosure of information obtained by the Health Service Commissioner or his officers in the course of or for the purposes of an investigation.

Common Law

In the medical context there is a long held presumption that a duty of confidence exists in the doctor-patient relationship. Until recently there was little by way of caselaw to support this. The general principles of this duty were laid out by Lord Goff in the 'spycatcher case' *Attorney –General- v-Guardian Newspapers Ltd (No2) [1990] 1AC 109* as follows: '…. A duty of confidence arises when confidential information comes to the knowledge of a person (the confidant) in circumstances where he had notice or is held to have agreed , that the information is confidential, with the effect that it would be just in all the circumstances that he should be precluded from disclosing the information to others…..'

The existence of this broad general principle reflects the fact that there is such a public interest in the maintenance of confidences, that the law will provide remedies for their protection……..Lord Goff

Unlawful use of patient information may attract a civil liability claim under breach of confidence and Art 8 of the Human Rights Act 1998 (respect for private life) or a complaint to the General Medical Council. In the case of *Pamela Cornelius –v- Dr Nicola de Tarants [2001] EMLR 329*, the claimant was awarded £300.00 for injury to feelings after a medicolegal expert passed a copy of her psychiatric report to the General Practitioner and a consultant Psychiatrist without her consent. Compensation can also be awarded under the Data Protection Act 1998 for breach arising out of the Act. If the information Commissioner rules that information is being used contrary to the Acts, an Enforcement notice can be issued against the Health Authority / organisation.

Contract

The duty of confidence can arise in a contractual relationship where this may be an express or implied term of the contract. Within the context of private medical care, where there is a contract between the patient and the doctor, there will be an express contractual term to maintain confidence. Outside of private treatment, there is no contractual relationship between the doctor and the patient within the NHS. However the doctor within the NHS has a contractual relationship with the employer. Under the contract of employment, there is an implied duty of fidelity or good faith. This is a duty of trust and confidence and consists principally of a number of aspects of confidentiality and non competition, some of which will apply after employment has ceased. The contractual obligation is that no employee shall breach their legal duty of confidentiality, allow others to do so or attempt to breach any of the employer's security systems or controls in order to do so. A doctor is in breach of his duty of fidelity if he uses or reveals patient information which by its very nature is confidential.

Exemptions from Confidentiality

A strict duty of confidence would create difficulties particularly in the transfer of information between medical professionals and therefore the patients' effective treatment may be jeopardised. The duty of confidence is not absolute and may be overridden by public interest. The law recognises that while a patient might have a personal interest in non disclosure, there may be a danger to others in doing so. The protection of confidence is a balancing act.

The remit of public interest and statutory exceptions to confidentiality will be explored with a caution that these exceptions should be invoked sparingly otherwise patients will cease to have confidence in the medical profession.

A. CONSENT

If a patient willingly consents, disclosure can be made by the health professional. Since the confidence is that of the patient, he is free to do whatever he wishes with the information. Having said that, the consenting patient must fully understand both the nature and the consequences of the disclosure i.e have sufficient information to make a decision. Consent to disclosure is preferably expressed but it may be implied.

Implied consent as a basic minimum, requires that a patient is at least aware of the practice of disclosure amongst other health professionals involved in their care. Reasonable effort must be made to bring the potential uses to the attention of patients. An example of implied consent as a basis for disclosure is when the patient is cared for by more than one medical team. There is a presumption that the patient consents to all the medical and nursing staff being informed for the continuity of care. Implied consent is also the remit under which patient information is used for risk management, audit, incident reporting and teaching purposes.

Implied consent is not without its difficulties and therefore strongly advised to obtain a written consent to disclosure. Where the information is anonymised, the consent of the patient can be dispensed with. (R-v-Dept of Health exp Source Informatics Ltd [2002] 2 WLR 940

B. PUBLIC INTEREST

The need to have a medical matter remain confidential is a public interest. Disclosure in public interest is a balancing exercise between the two interests : protection of the public and protection of the patient. This was succinctly expressed by Lord Gott in *A-G-v-Guardian Newspaper (No2) [1988] 1 All ER 545*'...although the basis of the laws protection of confidence is that there is a public interest that confidences should be preserved and protected by the law, nevertheless, that public interest may be outweighed by some other countervailing public interest which favours disclosure'.

The following are grounds for disclosure based on public interest:

I. Risk to Health and Safety of Others

This proviso is well illustrated with case law in the leading case of W-v- Egdell (1990) 1All ER 835, (1989) 4 BMLR 96(CA).

Facts of the case:

The plaintiff was imprisoned in a secure hospital following conviction for killing and other violent crimes. He made an application to a tribunal for transfer to a regional unit as a step towards release into the community. Dr Egdell was sought to give independent psychiatrist opinion. He felt that the plaintiff was still a danger to the public. W's case was withdrawn and the case was to be reviewed under the Mental Health Act 1983. Dr Egdell's report would not have been included in the reports reviewed by the tribunal under this process. Dr Egdell felt that this report should be considered and sent a copy to the medical director of the secure hospital and also the Home Office.

W brought an action for breach of confidence. At the first instance, the court found for the defendant as the breach was justified as being in public interest. W appealed. The Court of Appeal dismissed the appeal.

Lord Justice Bingham stated :

The parties were agreed as I think rightly , that the crucial question was how, on the special facts of the case, the balance should be struck between the public interest in maintaining professional confidences and the public interests in protecting the public against possible violence. Only the most compelling circumstances could justify the doctor acting in a way which would injure the immediate interests of his patient, as the patient perceived them, without obtaining his consent.

The judge preferred to rest his conclusion on a broader ground which was in effect that rarely, disclosure may be justified on the ground that it is in the public interest, which, in certain circumstances such as, for example investigation by the Police of a grave or very serious crime, might override the doctors duty to maintain his patients' confidence.

Given the courts acceptance of the fact that confidence may be breached in the public interest , there are limitations to the extent of disclosure. Guidance on this is laid out in the above case by LJ Bingham. He makes clear that the disclosure may be made:

CONFIDENTIALITY

a. Only to those whom it is necessary to tell so as to protect the public interest. The 'need to know' basis is also reiterated by the GMC guidance 'Confidentiality: Protecting Patients & Providing Information' (2004) para 36, and guidance document by the Department of Health 'The Protection and Use of Patient Information (1990).

b. To justify disclosure the risk must be real rather than fanciful. '..only the most compelling circumstances could justify a doctor acting in a way which could injure the immediate interests of his patient as the patient perceives them without his consent'.

c. More specifically, this real threat must involve a risk of physical harm, as opposed to some form of harm. The degree of harm that would come to the third party unless confidence is disclosed is a most important factor when determining whether disclosure is justified in public interest. The more probable and the more serious the magnitude of harm in question, then the more likely that the courts will hold that the disclosure to be in the public interest.

Other circumstances where disclosure may be justified in public interest of risk to health and safety of others include:

i. Driving when medically unfit and unsafe- disclosure can be made to DVLA.

ii. Serious communicable disease - The health care professional may disclose information to other health care professionals responsible for the care of the patient or to the patient's sexual partner/ spouse, that is specific identifiable individuals who are at risk of infection . The disclosure can be made only after the patient has been counselled by the medical team involved in his care and the patient has refused to give consent. (GMC: Serious Communicable Diseases. (1997))

iii. Neglect or abuse in a minor or incompetent. Section 47 of the Children's Act 1989 empowers professionals to share information where children are at risk of significant harm without obtaining the consent of the parent. It is however best practice to inform the parent of the decision to share information about them where possible (except where this would place the child at further risk). Guidance about sharing information in such cases can be obtained from the designated child protection officer . The GMC in its guidance 'Confidentiality :.... .....' (April 2004) states that 'disclosure should only be made without the patient's consent if the patient is unable to give consent and such disclosure is in the patients interest'

(para 38, 39).

II. Prevention and Detection of Crime

The public interest justification will support disclosure to prevent or detect serious crime and facilitate the due process of the criminal justice system. ' ...where a disclosure may assist in the prevention , detection or prosecution of a serious crime'. (GMC : Confidentiality: Protecting and Providing Information (para 37).

Similarly the Department of Health guidance on disclosure for the prevention of serious crime states that passing on information to help tackle serious crime ....may be justified if the following conditions are satisfied:

i. Without disclosure the task of preventing, detecting or prosecuting the crime would be seriously prejudiced or delayed

ii. Information is limited to what is strictly relevant to a specific investigation

iii. There is satisfactory undertaking that the information will not be passed to or used for any purpose other than the present investigation

III. Teaching and Research

Disclosure of patient information may be essential for the conduct of medical research, teaching and clinical audit. The justification for this exception to confidentiality recognises the public interest in properly conducted research and learning. GMC guidance on this is stated in 'Confidentiality' (2004)

' ....In these circumstances you should still obtain patients' express consent to the use of identifiable data or arrange for members of the health care team to anonymise records.' (para 15-18)

In the case of anonymised data, consent of the patient is not needed. This was established in the case *R-v-Dept of Health ex parte Source Informatics Ltd [2000] 2WLR 940*.

Facts of the case:

The Dept of Health argued that it was a breach of confidence to use anonymised data by the American Company, Source Informatics Ltd. Source Informatics replied that it was not, using one of its main arguments the fact that the patient would remain anonymous. The Appeal Court rightly concluded that there was no breach of confidence by the use of patient anonymised data.

Lord Justice Simon Brown said that 'the patient has no proprietary claim to the prescription form or to the information it contains. Of course he can bestow or withhold his custom as he pleases. But that gave the patient no property in the information and no right to control its use provided only and always that his privacy is not put at risk...'

The Department of Health has provided additional guidance in the document Local Research Ethics Committee HSG 91(5). Some of its recommendations are as follows:

- No individual should be recognisable from research without their explicit consent and the information should be destroyed when it is no longer needed.

- Where a situation arises where it would be impracticable to seek a patient's consent, the Local Research &Ethics Committee (LREC) must be satisfied that the research is in public interest, albeit that if the patient has indicated that he does not want his records released, this should be respected.

- Information should not be obtained without the consent being obtained from the health care professional and no approach should be made to the patient without the consent of the healthcare professional responsible for his care.

Approval of a research project by the LREC does not justify disclosure of patient information. The Dept of Health guidance to Research Ethics Committee is detailed in HSG (91)(5) para 3. These guidelines begin from a premise that the research subject's consent is required to disclosure.

IV. Clinical Risk Management and Audit

The Data Protection Act 1998 identifies circumstances in which use and disclosure of health information without express consent is permissible. A pragmatic approach is whether it is reasonably practicable to obtain express consent. Whilst this may not be always possible, consideration should be given to anonymised data. If consent cannot be obtained and the data anonymised, one has to weigh it up on whether it is in public interest. This is highly likely to weigh in the direction of using the data bearing in mind the importance of Clinical Risk Management to the Clinical Governance agenda and patient care.

The test suggested by the Information Commission is whether the use of the information that is necessary for medical purposes can be achieved with a 'reasonable degree of ease' without using information capable of identifying individual patient. (The Information Commission Guidance- Use and Disclosure of Health Data (May 2002). Justification can also be based on interests of protecting health and /or public safety (pressing social need) within the meaning of Art 8 of the European Convention of Human Rights. The disclosure must be proportionate to the aim intended i.e. minimalist use of the information.

C. STATUTORY DISCLOSURE

Earlier in this chapter we have seen how the law imposes a duty of confidentiality on the holder of patient information. The law through legislation may also modify that duty of confidentiality, in a given set of circumstances imposing a duty to disclose certain confidential information. The following legislation require disclosure to be made as a matter of law:

- Public Health (Control of Disease) Act 1984 supplemented by Public Health (Infectious Diseases) Regulations 1988 (SI 1988/1546)

  Section 11(1) of the Act provides that a registered medical practitioner shall send to the appropriate officer notice of any patient with a notifiable disease (s10 a-e)

- National Health Service (Venereal Diseases) Regulations 1974 (SI1974/29)

  Provides for the disclosure to a medical practitioner or to a person employed under the direction of a medical practitioner information about persons suffering from a sexually transmitted disease for the purpose of treatment and prevention.

- Abortions Regulations 1991 (SI 1991, No 499)

  Para 4(1) of the Regulations provides for disclosure of termination of pregnancy and information relating to the termination to the appropriate Clinical Medical Officer.

- The Health and Social Care Act 2001

  Section 60 of this Act empowers the secretary of state to authorise the use of patient information for medical purposes without the patient's consent where the person or organisation applying for this authorisation can show there is no practical alternative.

- The Health Service (Control of Patient Information) Regulation 2002

  (SI 2002, No 1438).

  This makes it lawful for cancer registries and the Public health laboratory service to collect and use identifiable patient information for authorised purposes. Para 2 of the Regulations allows for the use of confidential information relating to patients for the diagnosis or treatment of neoplasia to be processed for medical purposes. This includes the surveillance and analysis of health and diseases, the monitoring and audit of health and health related care, provision and outcomes where such provision have been made for health and health related care, medical research approved by the LREC. (para 2 (1) a-d)

- Misuse of Drugs Act 1971

  Misuse of Drugs (Notification of & Supply to Addicts Regulations 1973)

  (SI 1973/799)

  These pieces of legislation allows the Secretary of State to serve notice to any doctor or pharmacist requiring him to furnish such particulars as may be so specified relating to the quantities in which and the number and frequency of the occasions on which these drugs were prescribed, administered or supplied by him.

- NHS (Notification of Births & Deaths) Regulations 1982 (SI 1982/286)

Provides for the statutory disclosure of births and deaths records to the appropriate Registry.

- Police and Criminal Evidence Act 1984

Section 9 of the Act allows for special access to what is termed excluded material for the purposes of a criminal investigation, but only after a warrant from the courts. Section 17 allows access to personal records which relate to an individual's physical or mental health.

D. COURT PROCEEDINGS

In the course of legal proceedings, a health professional may be ordered to give evidence or disclose information about his patient. The courts' overriding objective is to ensure justice by balancing the need to keep the patient's confidence and allowing disclosure of relevant information.

During the 'Disclosure ' stage in civil litigation, the parties to the action must disclose information which has a bearing on the case or a party intends to rely on. Where disclosure involves a patient's medical records, consent of the patient is required even before disclosure to his legal team. Any limitation placed on the extent of disclosure must be respected. There is no duty to disclose a patient's records simply because the courts have given directions for 'Disclosure'. The consent of the patient must be obtained. The health professional is only obliged to make disclosure only if ordered to do so personally by the court. This will be in the form of a court order or a witness summons to give evidence in court. The justification for this being in connection with legal proceedings and the administration of justice. (Data Protection Act 1998 sch 3 para 6(a); 7(1)(a).

PARTICULAR PROBLEMS

- Duty to young patients and those who may lack competence:

Incompetent patients, children and young people under the age of 16 years have the same rights to confidentiality as any other client. If disclosure is requested,

the patient child or incompetent adult cannot give consent. Consent is therefore obtained from the appropriate person or authority, parents or those with parental responsibility if the disclosure is necessary and in the patient's best interest.

In the case of a young person (13 – 16years) who is deemed competent, any disclosure should be based on the child's ability to understand the nature and consequences of the disclosure.

Ethical and legal obligations arise where a child/young person may be a victim of neglect or abuse by the parent / carer. The Children Act 1989 and related legislation impose a statutory obligation on a number of professionals such as teachers and healthcare professionals to report actual or suspected harm to children. 'If you believe a patient to be a victim of neglect or physical, sexual or emotional abuse and that the patient cannot give or withhold consent to disclosure, you should give information promptly to an appropriate responsible person or statutory agency , where you believe that the disclosure is in the patient's best interests……..'

(GMC: Confidentiality:…….(2004)

- Duty to a deceased

Death does not end the duty of confidentiality to the patient. Information relating to the deceased medical records should be disclosed only to someone who is the deceased's executor or personal representative. Evidence of this status must be obtained and retained in the records before disclosure.

- Duty to Third Parties

In English Law it is still very much the position that one person will not usually be held liable for harm done by another person. The public interest justification for disclosure does not impose a new duty on the doctor to disclose information to a third party at risk of harm. Only where the health carer exercises some degree of control over the patient may a duty be imposed. This latter case is particularly relevant to doctors in psychiatry. It is likely that English Courts will take the view that where a doctor who exercises control over an individual can reasonably foresee that the individual's action will harm identifiable third party , then a duty can arise to warn the third party.

PATIENT ACCESS TO MEDICAL RECORDS

This section aims to set out the relevant guidance and legal obligations of doctors in relation to the patient's access to their medical records. Disclosure to patients can be formal or informal. Informal disclosures commonly occur in the clinic or inpatient setting where the patient requests to see a copy of a document in their files. In the Obstetric setting, access is the norm as the patients carry their own notes.. Formal requests for access to records is best referred to the designated Records Officer for the hospital for appropriate processing.

The legal framework that underpin access to health records by patients are as follows:

A. Data Protection Act 1998

All manual and computerised medical records about living patients can be accessed under this Act. Patients have a right of access to health records which:

- are about them and from which they can be identified
- consists of information relating to their physical or mental health or condition and
- have been made by or on behalf of a health professional in connection with their care.

The Act applies to all records regardless of when they were created. Generally any competent adult or their agents can apply for access under this Act. Parents may access on behalf of their children if it is in the best interests of the child. Similarly a person with an Enduring Power of Attorney or persons appointed by the courts to manage the affairs of an incompetent patient may obtain access in their best interests.

If access is by a third party it is essential to obtain proof that the third party is acting on the patient's behalf with the consent of the patient.

Limitations to access

Within the Data Protection Act 1998, there are limitations imposed on access by patients to their medical records. These limitations can be overridden by a court order or if it is necessary to establish or defend a legal right. They are as follows:

- Disclosure may be denied to some or all the records if in the opinion of the appropriate health professional, it is likely to cause serious harm to the patient or other persons.

- In *R-v- Midglamorgan FHSA exp Martin (1995)*, access was refused on grounds that disclosure might be detrimental to the applicant who had a history of psychological problems. The Court of Appeal held that a health professional could deny a patient access to his records if it was in the patient's best interest to do so. There is no absolute right of access to medical records.

- Records or parts of it which identify a third party whose consent has not been obtained cannot be disclosed except where the third party is a health professional. This is relevant for example where a couple undergo tests for infertility under the records of the woman and subsequently the woman requests access to her medical records. As the man is not a party to the access, any records that will identify him must not be disclosed without his consent unless it is reasonable to dispense with it. (Data Protection Act s7(4))

- Records which have the status of legal professional privilege may not be disclosed.

- Information on the storage of gametes /embryo that identifies whether an individual was or may have been born as a result of Assisted Conception Techniques may not be disclosed.

- Disclosure of adoption records or court orders under the Child Act 1989 (care order, contact order, supervision order) may not be disclosed.

B. Medical Reports Act 1988

The applies to access to employment or insurance medical reports and puts an obligation on the authors of the medical report and those who seek to access the reports. This Act is particularly important to medical practitioners and occupational physicians who are involved in the care of the patient and write a report on suitability of a job in relation to the patient's health or for insurance companies. Medical reports written by experts or any medical practitioner who has never been involved in the care of the patient are excluded from the Act.

The consent of the patient to whom the report applies must be obtained before a request for a medical report is complied with. The author of the report must be satisfied that the patient has consented to the release of the information.

British Medical Association policy is 'that doctors should refuse to complete a medical report for insurance or employment purposes unless satisfied that the following criteria are met :

- a written informed consent has been given
- a separate copy of the consent is provided for the retention of the author of the report.
- the request for medical information comes from the company's medical officer appropriately designated to carry out such functions.

The GMC provides further guidance on this in 'Confidentiality:.....' para 33-35:

The employer or insurance company requesting the medical report must inform the patient of his rights under the Access to Medical Report Act as follows :

- to refuse consent to the release of the medical report
- to have access to the report before or after it is sent to the applicant.
- after seeing the report before it is sent, to instruct the doctor not to send the report
- to request an amendment of the report
- if the patient wishes to see the report, the doctor must not dispatch it to the applicant for 21days, allowing the patient time to have access and until the patient has indicated his willingness to release the report.

Whether the patient sees the report before or after it is sent, he is entitled to receive a copy of the report. The doctor may charge a reasonable fee for supplying a copy of the report. A patient has a continuing right to access the report up to six months after it has been sent. Therefore the doctor must have a copy retained for at least six months.

C. Access to Health Records Act 1990

The Act provides a right of access to the manual records of deceased patients made since 1/11/91. (The DPA 1998 does not apply to deceased patients' records). Any person with a claim arising from the death of a patient has a right of access to information covered by the Act and directly relevant to that claim.

An executor or dependants of the deceased can therefore apply for access.

Access may be denied:

a. if in the opinion of the health professional it is likely to cause serious harm to somebody's physical or mental health;
b. the patient gave the information on the understanding that it would be kept confidential. Therefore no information at all can be disclosed if the patient requested absolute confidentiality.
c. the records identifies a third party whose consent has not been obtained unless that person is a health professional who has cared for the patient.

D. Freedom of Information Act 2000

The Act gives the public a right to access information held by public authorities which includes the NHS. Members of the public can make a request for disclosure about matters such as staffing levels, resource allocation, spending, risk management policies, outcome of investigations to adverse incidents, complaints and individual professional performance. It does not give access to patient's health records which is already covered by the Data Protection Act 1998. There are exemptions to disclosure of information if it relates to personal information of staff, court records and pending investigations.

The Act should be seen as an integral part of the governance agenda - openness, accountability, informed choice and a patient focused NHS.

SUMMARY

This chapter has shown how the common law, statutes and professional obligations interplay in a similar but different approach to protect a patient's right to confidentiality and access to medical records.

- There is a prima facie right of the individual to confidence of their medical records.
- Confidentiality is a legal obligation, a requirement established within professional codes of conduct.
- All NHS bodies and those carrying out functions on their behalf have a common law duty of confidentiality to patients and a duty to maintain professional, ethical standards of confidentiality.
- The duty of confidentiality is not absolute. Disclosure may be justified in the public interest.
- The duty of confidence does not apply to fully anonymised data.
- The duty of confidence does not attach to information in the public domain.
- Any disclosure of patient information with a health professional must be in the course of duty. You must make sure that anyone to whom you disclose personal information understands that it is given to them in confidence, which they must respect. Anyone receiving personal information in order to provide care is bound by a legal duty of confidence, whether or not they have contractual or professional obligations to protect confidentiality.
- Discussion with relatives must be with the patient's consent. In the case of an incompetent patient, only if this is in their best interests.
- Conversations relating to confidential matters affecting patients should not take place in situations where they may be overheard by passers-by.
- Requests for disclosure of patient records or access by the patient must be referred to the appropriate staff in the organisation designated to deal with such matters.
- If disclosure is authorised by the patient, the records should only be released to the patient or appropriate person or authority.

CONFIDENTIALITY

- You must be satisfied that there are appropriate arrangements for the security of personal information when it is stored, sent or received any electronic means.
- Any breach of confidentiality may be regarded as misconduct or gross misconduct which may be subject to disciplinary action.

References
1. General Medical Council:
   - Good Medical Practice (May 2001)
   - Confidentiality : Protecting and Providing Information (2004)
   - Serious communicable diseases
2. British Medical Association:
   Confidentiality and disclosure of health information. London BMA 1999
   Guidelines on the Access to Medical Reports Act 1988 : London BMA 1988

3. Department of Health: Protecting and Using Patient Information . A manual for Caldicott guardians. www.gov.uk/assetRoot/04/06/81/36/04068136.pdf
4. Confidentiality: NHS Code of Practice, Dept of Health 2003. www.doh.gov.uk/ipu/confiden/

Statutes
1. Data Protection Act 1998
2. Access to Medical Reports Act 1988
3. Access to Health Records Act 1990
4. Data Protection Act 1998
5. Misuse of Drugs Act 1971
6. Police and Criminal Evidence Act 1984
7. Human Fertilisation and Embryology Act 1990
8. Health Act 1999
9. Health Service Commissioners Act 1993
10. Public Health (Control of Diseases) Act 1984
11. Health and Social Care Act 2001
12. Human Rights Act 1998
13. Freedom of Information Act

Statutory Instruments
1. Abortions Regulations 1991
2. NHS (Venereal Diseases) Regulations 1974
3. NHS Trusts (Venereal Diseases) Directions 1991
4. NHS (Notification of Births & Death) Regulations
5. The Health Service (Control of Patient Information) Regulation 2002

Case law
1. Attorney General-v- Guardian Newspapers Ltd (1990) 1 AC 109
2. Fraser-v-Evans [1969] 1QB 349, CA
3. MS-v- Sweden (1997) 45 BMLR 133 (ECHR)
4. Pamela Cornelius –v- Dr Nicola de Tarants [2001] EMLR 329
5. R-v- Dept of Health exp Source Informatics Ltd [2002] 2WLR 940
6. W-v-Egdell (1990) 1AllER 835, (1989) 4 BMLR 96 (CA)

Chapter 6
END OF LIFE DECISIONS

This chapter has been inspired and included in the light of the recent judicial review application brought by Mr Oliver Burke against the General Medical Council (GMC) and subsequent appeal by the GMC setting aside the high court declaration that the GMC guidance on withholding and withdrawing life prolonging treatment was unlawful. The high court in the first instance found that an advance directive to require artificial nutrition and hydration (ANH) could be valid and that a number of the GMC guidance was unlawful. That decision was overruled at the appeal.

This case illustrates the ethical and legal challenges faced by clinicians in making end of life decisions. It is not intended in this chapter to explore the difficult albeit sensitive scenarios that arise at the end of life but to outline the legal principles and professional guidance and ethical safeguards that underpin the decision making.

This chapter will be discussed under the following headings:

a. Withholding and withdrawing life prolonging treatment
b. Do Not Resuscitate orders
c. Advance Directives

WITHOLDING AND WITHDRAWING LIFE PROLONGING TREATMENT

The ultimate aim of medical treatment is to provide benefit for the patient and treatment should not be prolonged if that cannot be achieved. As medical technologies continue to provide treatment options to prolong life despite organ failure there becomes a marked blurring of the dividing line between life and death. An important distinction must be made between withdrawal of treatment when it is futile and confers no benefit, and active intentional termination of life.

The House of Lords laid down the principles relating to withholding or withdrawing life prolonging treatments: (a) that it is lawful and (b) medical decisions for the incompetent patient should be made by the doctors in the best interest of the patient. *(Airedale NHS Trust –v- Bland [1993] AC 189)*

Facts of the case

Anthony Bland was in a persistent vegetative state for three and half years with no prospect of recovery. The Health Authority sought a declaration that it would be lawful to withdraw and withhold life prolonging treatment. The House of Lords held it to be lawful if it was not in the patient's best interests that his life should be prolonged.

When a patient is close to death the purpose of care is to ease the process of death and in those circumstances it is acceptable to withhold or withdraw life prolonging treatment. The decision might be considered where there is brain death, persistent vegetative state and the 'no chance situation' where treatment simply delays death without ant alleviation of suffering This does not apply to oral feeding and hydration but medical treatment of which artificial nutrition and hydration (ANI I) are inclusive.

When is court approval required ?

Doctors treating terminally ill patients or patients in persistent vegetative state often have to approach end of life decisions and the ethical, moral and legal issues that arise with those decisions. In practice these decisions are made sensitively, judiciously with reasoned clinical acumen in the best interests of the patient . Whilst many cases will be decided between the medical team and those closest to the patient, in particularly difficult and contentious cases, the courts are asked to decide. The High Court has jurisdiction to make declarations as to the best interests of an adult who lacks decision-making capacity. This jurisdiction will be exercised when there is an important legal or ethical issue e.g. withdrawal or continuance of medical treatment.

1. Persistent Vegetative State

As a matter of good practice and the law, court approval is required in these clinical conditions. The House of Lords in the Bland case upheld a declaration that it would be lawful to withhold life prolonging treatment and care from the patient as being in the best interests peaceably to die; whereas continuing treatment would have been futile. In Scotland the court does not require each PVS case to come before it to withdraw treatment.

2. Contentious Cases

Approval of the court is required in patients who are not in PVS where there is contention over the prognosis and or best interests with the relatives of the patient or where an Advance Directive (AD) stipulates treatment in circumstances where medical evidence shows that it is futile. The case of the severely damaged baby Charlotte which was widely reported in the national newspapers in 2005 is an example of such. The case if Glass -v- U.K [2004] 1FLR 1019 in the European Courts of Human Rights(ECHR) illustrates the value of court approval when there is a dispute.

Facts of the case:

The parents of an 11 year old child challenged the decision of the medical team to provide the child with palliative care rather than aggressive medical treatment. The child was removed from the care of the hospital amidst a lot of strife and acrimony between the medical team and the parents. The parents sought a judicial review in the High Court after this but the High Court declined to intervene because the event in dispute had lapsed. The parents took the case to the ECHR alleging a breach of Art 8 (Right to a private life) of the Human Rights Convention. The ECHR found the U.K in breach of Art 8 because the NHS

Trusts had failed to obtain a declaration from the High Court as to the lawfulness of its decision.

Human Rights Implications:

Decisions to withdraw or withhold life prolonging treatment may encroach on the Human Rights Acts 1998. Health Authorities which are public bodies and hence health professionals are expected to ensure that medical decisions are compatible with the Act. The spirit of the Act is to promote human dignity and reflective decision making. Failure to comply with the Act could result in costly litigation and fines for the breach.

The provisions in the Act that are relevant to end of life decisions are:

- Article 2: The right to life

    - The withdrawal of artificial nutrition and hydration does not constitute an intentional deprivation of life within the meaning of Art 2.

    - The positive obligation on the state to provide life sustaining treatment is in the circumstances where such treatment is in the best interests of the patient.

    - Withdrawal of artificial nutrition and hydration from patients in PVS is compatible with the Human Rights Act 1998.(NHS Trust A- v- M, NHS Trust B-v- H [2001] 1FLR 406

- Article 3: To be free from inhuman & degrading treatment

    - There is no positive obligation upon a state under the ECHR to allow for euthanasia or assisted suicide.

    - Where treatment given offers no benefit to the patient or he or she will never have awareness or the reality to interact and is therefore unable to experience benefit, the duty to protect life must be balanced against the right to subject the patient to inhuman or degrading treatment.

- Art 8: To respect for privacy and family life
- Article 10: Freedom of expression, which includes the right to hold opinions and to receive information.
- Article 14: To be free from discriminatory practices in respect of these rights.

ADVANCE DIRECTIVE (A.D)

The guiding principle underlying the development of advance directives (A.D) is the right of the competent patient to autonomous decision making and choices. An A.D provides for forward planning and protection of the patient's dignity, and wishes in the event of incapacity. The ethical and legal principles that underpin patient decision making has been explored in the chapter on 'Consent'.

Advance Directives are not new in clinical practice. They have existed in advance refusal of blood transfusion by Jehovah's witness patients. What is new is the scope to which these advance decisions – acceptance or refusal of treatment and interventions can be applied to, even if those decisions result in the death of the patient or contrary to medical opinion.

An A.D can request specific treatment but particular problems may arise where an advance directive requests a particular treatment which is not in the best interests of the patient or conflicts with the health professional's clinical judgement, or contrary to public policy (such as excluding basic care to maintain bodily cleanliness, alleviate pain and suffering and provision of natural feeding or requesting euthanasia or assisted suicide).

An A.D must comply with the requirements of a valid consent i.e. the patient must have been competent when it was made, voluntarily and with a broad understanding of its implications. (see chapter on 'Consent') Therefore advance acceptance or refusals of medical treatment can be legally binding on health professionals if certain conditions are met. The common law lends support to the lawfulness of A.D in the case of *Re K (Medical Treatment : Consent) (2001).* The validity of an A.D came to be decided by the High Court. Hughes J stated ' It is ….. clearly the law that the doctors are entitled … to treat the patient if it is known that the patient, provided he was of sound mind and full capacity , has let it be known that he does not consent and that such treatment is against his wishes. To this extent an advance indication of the wishes of the patient of full capacity and sound mind are effective'.

Statutory backing in support of A.D is found in Part 1 section 24 of the Mental Capacity Act 2005 which sets out the requirement for validity and applicability as follows:

1. An advance decision does not affect the liability which a person may incur for carrying out or continuing a treatment in relation to the patient unless the decision is at the material time (a) valid and (b) applicable to the treatment.

2. An advance decision is not valid if the patient (a) has withdrawn the decision at a time when he had capacity to do so (b) has, under a lasting Power of Attorney created after the A.D was made, conferred authority on the donee to give or refuse consent to the treatment to which the A.D relates (c) has done anything which clearly is inconsistent with the A.D remaining his fixed decision.

3. A.D is not applicable to the treatment in question if at the material time the patient has capacity to give or refuse consent to it.

4. Any decision is not applicable to the treatment in question if (a) that treatment is not the treatment specified in the A.D (b) any circumstances specified in the AD are absent or (c) there are reasonable grounds for believing that circumstances exist which the patient did not anticipate at the time of the A.D and which would have affected his decision had he anticipated them.

5. An A.D is not applicable to life sustaining treatment unless

    a. the decision is verified by a statement by the patient to the effect that it is to apply to that treatment even if life is at risk,

    b. the decision and statement comply with subsection 6 below

6. A decision or statement complies with this subsection only if

    a. it is in writing

    b. It is signed by the patient or by another person in his presence and under his direction;

    c. The signature is made or acknowledged by the patient in the presence of a witness;

d. The witness signs it or acknowledges his signature in the patient's presence.

An A.D that is valid and relevant to the circumstances should be respected. Particular care has to be taken to ensure that the A.D. still obtains and that the anticipated event reflect those that arise bearing in mind the present circumstances, how long ago the A.D. was made. Where there is doubt, the course of action most likely to preserve life should be adopted.

DO NOT ATTEMPT RESUSCITATION ORDERS (DNAR)

It is clear to all doctors that there are some patients who have suffered a cardiac arrest for whom this event is the final in their dying process or terminal illness. Attempted resuscitation is therefore inappropriate, unlikely to be successful and if anything nature should be allowed to take its cause uneventfully. The decision of DNAR can raise ethical, legal and emotive issues for all concerned in certain circumstances. It is not intended here to identify the various clinical scenarios where this decision may arise, but to outline the legal and ethical principles that underpin the decision making. Mentally competent patients can make an advance direction to refuse cardiopulmonary resuscitation (CPR) which is effective provided it is valid and relates to the circumstance in time. Where the current DNAR status is unknown, there is a presumption in favour of resuscitation in the best interests of the patient that the potential benefit outweighs the burden.

A 'DNAR' decision should be seen as part of the forward planning of patient care in those who have an advance direction to that effect and those patients whose condition indicates that effective CPR is unlikely to be successful. The courts have confirmed that it is lawful to withhold CPR on the basis that it would not confer a benefit upon the patient where considerations has been given to the relevant medical factors and to whether the treatment may provide a reasonable quality of life. (Re R (adult : Medical Treatment) [1990] 2FLR 99)

Framework For Decision Making

- Information

    Written information about CPR should be readily available to patients, relatives and those closest to them. This should include an explanation of the procedure, how decisions are made and the chances of a successful outcome. This information should be made available in a sensitive manner to competent patients with a terminal illness or where there is a foreseeable risk of cardiopulmonary arrest. Similarly in incompetent patients or children, persons close to them or those with parental responsibility respectively should be offered such information.

- Exploration

    Whenever a DNAR decision is contemplated by the medical team, wherever possible there should be a sensitive exploration with the patient or their close relatives of their wishes regarding CPR. Timely support and sensitive advance discussion should be initiated and encouraged by the responsible consultant or the most senior doctor with a senior nurse on duty. With children who lack competence, a decision should be reached with the parents or those with parental responsibility. Particular care needs to be taken in making this decision with competent children who can consent to medical treatment but their refusal can be overridden by a person with parental responsibility or the health professional.

- Clinical Issues
    - Decisions must be based on the individual patient's circumstances and reviewed regularly in the light of the patients clinical progress and wishes
    - Decision should be made judiciously guided by current guidelines and evidence based practice.
    - The decision should be guided by the overall benefit to the patient which must outweigh the burdens.
    - A realistic view must be given of the chances of survival.

- In an emergency where there is no advance decision, CPR should be attempted unless the patient is clearly in the terminal phase of illness or the burdens of treatment outweigh the benefits

- Responsibility

    Discussions of the advisability or otherwise of CPR should be undertaken by senior members of the medical and nursing team involved in the care of the patient and reach a consensus. This facilitates the effective communication of the decision to the relevant health professionals. The consultant takes overall responsibility for the decision. In the absence of the consultant, the next most senior member of the medical team in consultation with the most senior nurse will make the decision. This must be communicated to the lead consultant at the earliest opportunity who takes overall responsibility for this decision.

- Communication
    - Discussions about whether or not to attempt CPR and any advance directives must be entered in the clinical notes with the name of the doctor, dated, timed and signed.
    - DNAR decisions must be must be similarly entered in the clinical and nursing records.
    - The reason(s) for the DNAR order must be given and a time limit applied or not time limited in patients with terminal malignant disease.
    - The DNAR order should be communicated to the patient (who wants to know) and where the patient lack competence, people close to them.
    - Where a patient declines a discussion on CPR and such an order is made, this must be documented in the notes.

END OF LIFE DECISIONS

- Legal Issues
    - Decisions about CPR must be compatible with the Human Rights Act
    - Patients or relatives cannot insist on CPR which the healthcare team judges to be inappropriate but every effort should be made to accommodate wishes and preferences.
    - Relatives do not have the power of proxy to make decisions on behalf of a patient, unless they have a valid Power of Attorney. They can neither give or withhold consent for the patient.
    - Competent young people must be offered the opportunity to participate in the decision making.
    - With children who lack capacity the decision should be reached with those with parental responsibility.
    - In Scotland, people over 16 years can appoint a proxy decision maker who has the legal power to give consent to medical treatment when the patient loses capacity. (Adults with Incapacity (Scotland) Act)
    - Where a patient makes an advance directive not to be resuscitated their competence must be assessed carefully for the validity of the refusal.
    - Where there is serious disagreement between the patient, close relatives and the medical team legal advice should be sought early. In some cases, a court declaration may be needed.

FUTURE DEVELOPMENTS

Legislative guidance for end of life decisions which is currently guided by the common law is long overdue. The long awaited **Mental Capacity Act 2005** will provide the statutory framework for incompetent patients and end of life issues. It aims to give people the power to influence the type of care they want in the future and ensure that their wishes are carried out. It therefore builds on current law that already allows an appointed person to take care of an individuals financial affairs if they no longer have the ability to do so independently.

It recognises the role of proxy decision makers appointed by the patient and sets out a framework for acting and making decisions on behalf of adults 16 years and over, with clear guidance on the remit of Advance Directives.

References

1. GMC: Witholding and Withdrawing Life-prolonging Treatments: Good Practice in Decision-making.(2002)
2. Assessment of Mental Capacity: Guidance for Doctors and Lawyers: The Law Society (BMA 1995)
3. Witholding or Withdrawing Life Saving Treatment in Children: 'A framework for practice', Royal College of Paediatrics and Child Health, London 1997
4. Decision Relating to Cardiopulmonary Resuscitation: A joint statement from the British Medical Association, The Resuscitation Council (U.K) and the Royal College of Nursing.
5. Resuscitation Council (UK). Resuscitation guidelines 2000. London: Resuscitation Council (UK) , 2000

Chapter 7
CLINICAL GOVERNANCE

The words Clinical Governance (CG) and Risk Management (RM) are often flirted with by healthcare professionals with a miniscule understanding of the concept. It has become a very popular interview question and a threatening way to get doctors to boring meetings. A considerable number of the medical staff have no concept of partnership or ownership in the agenda, delegating it to the 'managers'. This is partly due to a lack of understanding, bogged down by paper work, malicious reporting and blame. 'If CG is not understood, viewed positively and implemented by staff, it is unlikely to be successful'. (Goodman, 1998).

In this chapter, I hope to bring knowledge and understanding to the agenda and a positive attitude to its implementation by medical staff.

ORIGIN:
CG was introduced in 1997 as a comprehensive framework to reduce risk and improve the quality of healthcare in the NHS. It has been prompted by failings in NHS organisations that have resulted in adverse incidents, inquiries and litigation. The development of Clinical Governance is designed to consolidate, codify and universalise often fragmented and far from clear policies and approaches by NHS organisations to govern the delivery of clinical services. It has developed incrementally and positively as a way of addressing concerns about the quality of care, with

a greater focus on patient safety than ever before. It has helped NHS organisations develop clearer lines of accountability and strengthen their risk management policies.

CG can be viewed as a whole system of cultural change which provides the means of developing the organisational capability to deliver sustainable, accountable, patient focused quality assured care. CG is an opportunity to find ways to move people out of the comfort zone of the status quo towards a more challenging culture where there is active learning and questions are asked in the spirit of learning and development. The overall objective of the CG strategy is to improve the quality of care given to patients, maintenance of a safer environment for patients, employees and visitors, and to reduce the NHS's losses to a minimum.

The main principles of CG are:
- clear lines of responsibility and accountability for the overall quality of clinical care;
- a comprehensive programme of quality improvement systems including clinical audit, evidence based practice, implementing clinical standards and guidelines, workforce planning and development;
- education and training ;
- clear policies aimed at managing risk;
- an integrated procedures for all professional groups to identify and remedy poor performance.

(www.doh.gov.uk/pricare/clingov.htm)

DEFINITION:
There is a plethora of definitions in the literature for CG. This reflects the ubiquitous nature of CG and its wide ranging application in all areas of healthcare and efforts to develop an understanding of the agenda. Common to all definitions of CG is the notion of an integrated approach to achieve improvement in quality of care.

I. 'A framework through which NHS organisations are accountable for continually improving the quality of their services and safeguarding high standards of care by creating an environment in which excellence in clinical care will flourish'

(Donaldson & Gray 1998)

This definition captures the provision of continuous quality improvement in the agenda.

II. 'A governance system for health care organisations that promotes an integrated approach towards management of inputs, structures and processes to improve the outcome of healthcare service delivery where health staff work in an environment of greater accountability for clinical quality'

This definition captures the management of inputs, structures, processes and outcomes as part of the CG agenda.

<u>Key players in the CG agenda</u>

- Staff
  The health service is a multitude of highly skilled, highly motivated, hard working and creative individuals. The staff of a healthcare organisation are crucial to how the challenges of CG can be met. CG is a chance to harness and value talents and skills of NHS staff and enhance performance through development of skills and knowledge. To do this, requires the drawing together of many strands of professional endeavour and management commitment into a cohesive programme of action in each healthcare organisation. Firstly, good recruitment, retention and development of staff will make a major contribution. Secondly, valuing staff is crucial to gain their support and create a positive work attitude, leadership and team. Thirdly, staff must participate in developing quality strategies and be encouraged to look critically at existing processes of care and improve them.

- Patients
  At the centre of CG must be a real partnership between patients and professionals. It is the patients who are the consumers and can best tell it 'as it really is'.

Professionals need to develop the mechanisms and the skills to listen with 'authentic curiosity' to patients. Only when we can see through the patients eyes, can we be confident that we are building into organisations and healthcare systems which are relevant for the patients at their centre.

The Components of Clinical Governance

The foundation:
Underpinning the successful implementation of CG is an awareness of the need for solid foundations to establish an enabling culture. CG demands new ways of working and thinking and changes in relationship between individuals, teams and organisation – <u>a change in culture</u>. There is a dependent relationship between achieving quality improvement and changing organisational culture. The organisational culture in which people work determines the clinical outcome and staff morale that prevails.

The foundation of the CG agenda requires an organisational culture where individuals and teams can openly discuss their practice (openness), reflect on what they do best and least, learn from mistakes (reflective practice) and value staff. CG will thrive best in an organisation that creates a working environment which is open and participative, where ideas and good practice are shared, where education and research are valued and where blame is used rarely. On the latter note we need to move towards a reflective non blame culture where 'what went wrong' not 'who went wrong' is the first response to a problem and where the same mistakes are not repeated by different people on a regular basis.

The importance of changing culture in order to achieve CG was recognised as the Dept of Health set out its vision for quality in the new NHS :........achieving meaningful and sustainable quality improvements, in the NHS requires a fundamental shift in culture, to focus effort where it is needed and to enable and empower those who work in the NHS to improve quality locally. (Secretary of State for Health , 1997)

The five cultural components described below identify the areas in which there is need to share beliefs, attitudes, values and norms of behaviour in order to deliver sustainable quality improvement in healthcare. (Davies et al,2000)

- Systems Awareness
  Healthcare organisations comprise myriad systems whose complex interactions can generate unplanned consequences. Most often, it is a system which fails, not a human. There is rarely a single causal element in a failure. When there is an untoward incident, the first response should always be to examine the systems involved. A culture which is system centred, identifies that human beings are fallible and errors are to be expected. It therefore focuses on factors influencing errors and remedial actions aimed at conditions at work.

- Team Work
  Modern healthcare has become increasingly complex, requiring co-ordinated and integrated systems of work. More and more, the interdependence of working methods demands partnership between clinicians, between clinicians and managers and between clinicians and patients. There is a strong association between good team work and the delivery of effective and innovative healthcare for patients. Team work is an essential first step in the success of the quality and safety agenda.

  'The days of quality improvement by exhortation have surely gone. We are in an era of partnership where team work will be the route to success and where we must specifically address the rough edges which stop organisations joining together to form genuine partnerships' (Donaldson 1998).

- Communication
  The CG agenda must be clearly defined and communicated to all staff to help them understand the relevance and their roles. Similarly information about audit results, organisational and practice changes must be promptly disseminated locally and easily available to all the staff. It requires an effective communication system.

- Ownership
  Ownership is about real participation of staff in all developments. It is about creating a working environment where structures are in place to support individuals so that professionals and teams are empowered to

own and therefore to solve problems

The idiom that people will support what they help to create is certainly true to advance and encourage the CG agenda.

- Leadership
Effective leadership is vital to the successful implementation of CG. Programmes for change are unlikely to be successful unless there is a consistent, unswerving commitment from the leaders to ensure that the programme acquires weight, credibility and staff support. It requires systems for accountability and responsibility at both the Trust and clinical level. At the Trust level, the medical director is the CG lead responsible for establishing, co-ordinating and managing the framework.

Each clinical speciality will identify a lead from within the department to take responsibility for and report at Trust level to the Medical Director who will feed into a select committee with responsibility for broader CG policies.

The Building blocks (key areas)

The key areas of CG can be subdivided into seven pillars.(Nicholls et al, 2000).

These correspond roughly to the areas of clinical audit, risk management, patient & public involvement, continuing professional development, clinical effectiveness, clinical information and staffing. NHS Trusts have a statutory obligation to maximise quality in these seven areas.

1. Clinical Effectiveness
The ethos is laid firmly on setting standards for clinical care guided by research evidence and monitoring it by clinical audit. Clinical effectiveness can be achieved when the best available clinical knowledge, evidence and information are made available to health professionals for planning, implementing and monitoring patient care. Clinical effectiveness helps to identify the rational for patient care as well as focusing on each clinician's professional accountability

to provide effective care. It is the interface between evidence based practice, risk management, quality improvement and clinical audit.

Defining quality and delivering clear and consistent service in health care means that increasingly, clinical decisions or health policy must be based on validated research evidence and approved guidelines. Clinical guidelines have been increasingly used as a tool to promote clinical effectiveness, improve clinical care and decrease variation in practice. It is the forum for implementation of evidence based practice which can facilitate significant improvements in clinical and other decision making and provide more efficient and cost effective health services. With care now being delivered by multidisciplinary teams, Integrated Care Pathways (ICP) have evolved and are used to determine 'locally agreed, multidisciplinary practice based on guidelines and evidence where available for a specific client group'.

2. Clinical Audit – is a quality improvement process that seeks to improve patient care and outcomes through systematic review of care against explicit criteria and the implementation of change. There is a contractual obligation on all staff to participate in regular clinical audit and review of clinical services. (Standards for Better Health).

Any clinical audit activity must be effectively managed to reflect and inform the CG agenda, improve safety and deliver significant improvement in the quality of care. Audit may evaluate provision/ organisation of services, process and outcome of care, changes in practice and benefits. Local audits should be linked to national audits such as those of NICE and the CHAI.

Clinical audit can be useful in :

- providing opportunities for training and education
- identifying and promoting good practice
- supporting more efficient use of resources
- improving working relationships and communication between staff, service users and other interested parties.

3. Continuing Professional Development
   Continuing professional development ensures that the best quality care within the healthcare is available by clinicians keeping up to date with current knowledge, learning new materials, practicing clinical skills with proficiency and developing new ones. To deliver care, healthcare organisations need to ensure that the staff they employ have the right skills, competence and appropriate training. To this end they must invest in training and development through continuing professional development and clinical supervision.

4. Staffing
   This is about having the right people with the right skills delivering the right care in the right place at the right time, with the aim of achieving the best outcomes. Each Health organisation should have a system for ensuring that medical staff are competent and supervised. A learning and development framework will enable staff have their learning needs identified and addressed. This framework should incorporate arrangements for learning and professional development based on the knowledge and skills framework, which defines and describes the knowledge and skills staff need to apply to their work and provide a consistent framework for review and development. The framework should encourage clinical teams and individuals to learn from what they do and improve matters as a result of that learning process. They also need to establish structures to ensure that educational and governance activities are properly coordinated and reflect the individual and service needs. Regular appraisals should be in place to help identify and bridge training gaps.

5. Patient Experience
   Patient and Public Involvement (PPI) is a crucial and integral component of CG. The agenda remains deficient unless the views of patients and public are sought and taken into account. They are the consumers of the health service and are best placed to comment on the quality of care they have received. PPI has the potential to improve the quality of policy and decision making; build relationships and confidence; ensure social, cultural and ethical considerations are included in decision and provide valuable insights

into why things go wrong . Patient involvement can be achieved through approaches that provide opportunities for involvement in decision making about their care, clear channels through which to voice their views, concerns and complaints, and a confidence that these will be acted upon.

Patients' and public perspective of care of services provide opportunities for reflection, new ideas and experiences that might not otherwise be known. The antiquated view of patients as passive recipients of care is no longer acceptable in a modern NHS. The involvement of the patient and the public is reflective of the maturity and openness of the NHS, and a key test of the effectiveness of arrangements for clinical governance. More than ever before, patients' and the public rightly expect involvement as consumers of public services. There is a statutory obligation on every NHS organisation to involve and consult patients and the public in the ongoing planning and provision of NHS services. (s11 Health & Social Care Act (2001)).

There are various approaches to inform and promote the PPI initiative. These include passive involvement through questionnaire surveys, in-depth interviews, observation or active involvement through focus groups and Performance Development Team (PDT). Similarly within Trusts', a number of structures have been developed to increase user and community involvement in the day to day running of the NHS:

a. Patient Advice and Liaison Service (PALS) – Provides confidential on the spot assistance to patients, service users, relatives, carers and staff using and working in the NHS.

b. Patient and Public Involvement Forums (PPI) – These are independent of the Trust and made up of volunteers in the local community who are enthusiastic about helping patients and members of the public to influence the way that local healthcare is organised and delivered.

c. Independent Complaints & Advocacy Service (ICAS) offers independent support to people wanting to make complaints about NHS services.

d. Overview & Scrutiny Committees (OSCS)- these are based in local authorities and have the power to review and scrutinise the local services as part of the wider agenda to seek health improvements and reduce health inequalities.

e. NHS Complaints Procedure- This has been reviewed to make it more accessible and ensure that complaints are dealt with speedily and efficiently. The emphasis is on listening to the service user to improve service and quality of care.

It is imperative that information from these sources are linked back to the organisation's governance committee to inform on quality of care and identify areas for improvement. Patient experience has the potential to improve the quality of policy and decision making, develop trust and demonstrate transparency and accountability. It broadens the perspective and insight of the organisation, avoid challenges and misunderstanding with the public by inclusion, understanding and real partnership.

6. Information

Effective communication is crucial to CG so that staff and public are well informed of the strategies in order to empower and encourage their involvement for CG to succeed. Each NHS organisation in drawing up how to work out the accountability details must ensure that they are communicated throughout the organisation.

7. Risk Management

This is principally concerned with the organisational strategies and framework within the organisation to manage risks. This is applied to both clinical and non clinical risks. At the organisational level, it focuses on the structures and processes for managing clinical and non clinical risks, to ensure that these are integrated with patient and staff safety, complaints and clinical negligence, and financial and environmental risk. A performance indicator for the risk management systems should be developed and monitored. The local risk management systems should be supported by the organisational risk management strategy, a pro active risk assessment which is fed into the organisation-wide risk assessment process and risk register.

SUMMARY

- Clinical Governance provides a framework to coordinate accountability, quality improvements and quality assurance efforts within an organisation.
- It is a framework for a range of activities that aims to promote, maintain and improve standards of patient care.
- It requires an organisation wide transformation, clinical leadership and a positive culture.
- It is about more than systems. It is about people, processes and culture.

Chapter 8
CLINICAL RISK MANAGEMENT

Clinical Risk Management (CRM) refers to the organisational systems or processes which aim to improve quality of healthcare, create and maintain safe systems of care. The diagram below illustrates its inter-relationship with other areas of the clinical governance agenda.

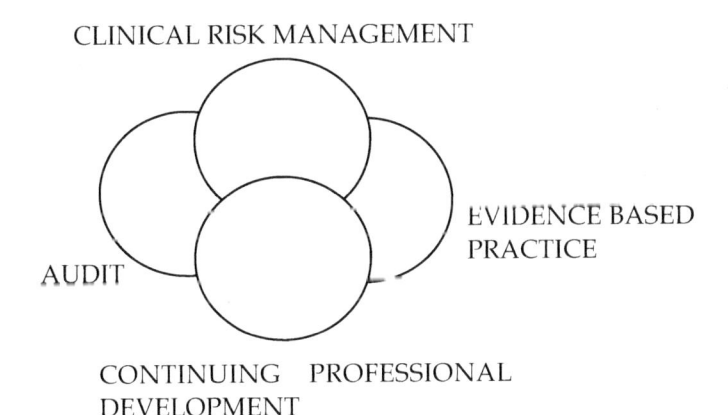

CLINICAL RISK MANAGEMENT

EVIDENCE BASED PRACTICE

AUDIT

CONTINUING PROFESSIONAL DEVELOPMENT

Definition:
Methods for the early identification of adverse events using either staff reports or systematic screening of records. This should be followed by creation of a database to identify common patterns and develop a system of accountability to prevent future incidents. (RCOG & Clinical Governance. London: RCOG 1999)

The drivers for CRM include the Clinical Governance agenda, reports and inquiries into adverse incidents leading to harm, the Clinical Negligence Scheme for Trusts (CNST) assurance standards (see Appendix E NHS Structures- NHSLA), complaints and litigation. A defensive and adversarial view of CRM focuses on litigation and cost containment. This distorted view deflects from the positive and robust view of improving well being of patients and quality of care. The latter view reflects the philosophy of using incident reporting to promote reflective practice and reduce the frequency of adverse events and harm to patients. The emphasis is on developing open and supportive frameworks to help organisations reflect upon their performance and learn from mistakes.

CRM is best managed within a framework that integrates all the aspects of clinical governance -clinical audit, clinical supervision, training and education, complaints and claim handling. At the organisational level it should be linked with other strategies and initiatives. The implementation of a risk management programme requires funding, a clear leadership for it and the development of a team/ coordinator to take day to day responsibility for incident reporting , data collection and audit. A successful CRM programme is achieved through carefully designed management systems with a positive organisational safety culture where incident reporting is viewed favourably without fear of punishment or detriment, teamwork, communication and user involvement.

The National Patient Safety Agency in its guide Seven Steps to Patient Safety describes the steps that NHS organisations should take to improve patient safety:

- Build a safety culture
- Lead and support staff
- Integrate the risk management activity
- Promote reporting
- Involve and communicate with patients and the public

- Learn and share safety lessons
- Implement solutions to prevent harm.

The Process for Managing Clinical Risk

Risk management approaches should aim to identify where risks occur in a system and solutions to reduce those risks. The former relies on the reporting mechanisms while the latter relies on systems analysis. To best utilise a CRM policy and ensure that adverse incidents do not or rarely occur, undertaking a thorough risk assessment is paramount.

Below is an outline of the process through which a clinical risk can be managed:

- Risk identification

   This aims to identify where an untoward incident / 'near miss' can or did occur. It can be retrospective examining the incident, 'where did things go wrong' or prospective scrutinising and analysing the existing system – 'what can go wrong' An incident is anything that a witness views worthy to address to eliminate a potential to cause harm. It would therefore contain a wide variety of occurrences such as unsafe conditions, unsafe behaviour, minor accidents that had the potential to be more serious, where a safety barrier was challenged and events where a potential environmental damage could result. A 'near-miss' is an event that signals a system weakness that if not remedied could lead to significant consequences in the future. As such a 'near-miss' is an opportunity to improve system structures and stability, and reduce risk exposure to potential catastrophe.

   The first stage of the risk assessment stage is incident reporting. A good incident reporting programme is the early warning system for potential complaints and claims. The reporting process must be quick, simple and staff must know whom to and how to report clinical incidents. All healthcare professionals have a professional and ethical responsibility to ensure patient safety, and reporting incidents is an integral part of that responsibility. There are also legal obligations to report incidents such as under the Health & Safety Act (Reporting of Injuries, Diseases and Dangerous Occurrences Regulations-RIDDOR), Medical Devices Agency (incidents involving medical devices, wheeled mobility equipment) the police (criminal activity) and the coroner (death within 24hours of admission, anaesthetic deaths).

When incidents are reported, causes can be identified and plans developed and implemented to prevent recurrence. The value of a risk identified is lost if management does not facilitate and encourage reporting of the incident. Hence management must create a culture of openness and learning where reporting is actively encouraged and there is no fear of disciplinary action. Incident reporting fails because it is given low priority, fear of reporting- blame, fear of writing statements and staff failure to identify serious incidents. The message that needs to be conveyed to health professionals is that incident reporting is actively wanted and non punitive. It is the cornerstone to learning from experience – a systematic approach to encourage learning and promote improvements in practice based on individual and aggregated analysis of incidents, complaints and claims.

At the national level, learning from experience through incident reporting is supported through the activities of the National Patient Safety Authority (NPSA). The NPSA is a special health authority that coordinates the effort of the National Health Service (NHS) to report incidents through the National Reporting and Learning System (NRLS).

- Root Cause Analysis (RCA)
Root Cause Analysis can be defined as a systematic investigation to the underlying causes and environmental context in which adverse incidents occur. It is a retrospective review of a patient safety incident undertaken in order to identify what, how and why it happened. The technique is used to investigate incidents in a thorough and rigorous way, promote a consistent approach to managing incidents and encourage learning. The analysis is then used to identify areas for change, recommendations and sustainable solutions, to help minimise the reoccurrence of the incident type in the future. RCA is the key to understanding the system errors involved in clinical incidents.

   a. In the analysis of an incident it is necessary to:

   b. Assess the direct and underlying root causes that enabled the incident

Determine corrective actions or solutions to rectify the root cause such that recurrence is much less likely.

Most events will have multiple causes that combine synergistically to produce the event. For RCA to be effective for human error analysis in healthcare, a range of factors must be considered, including individual, team, task, supervisory, management and policy influences. It should identify contributory factors that it may need to search for the underlying psychological causes. RCA provides the insights needed to develop effective error reduction strategies and solutions. Depending on the potential severity and complexity of the incident, determination of causes may be performed informally between the discloser and direct supervisor or may require an investigation team for a thorough analysis with subsequent recommendations.

The National Patient Safety Agency (NPSA) have developed an e-learning training package on RCA. The package provides NHS staff with guidance on how to analyse incidents, and an interactive tool to help them develop confidence in performing RCA. (www.npsa.nhs.uk/rca)

- Risk Control
  This can be undertaken using the following approaches:
  1. Solution Identification- this is aimed at minimising the risk subsequent to each cause and corrective actions that needs to be formulated. Ideally these corrective actions should eliminate the potential for recurrence, or reduce the potential impact in case of recurrence. The changes implemented must be carefully monitored and scrutinized to assess whether there are detracting factors such as cost, employee and management acceptance or new risk arising as a result of the changes.
  2. Resolution – It is intrinsic to the success of a CRM programme to ensure that the issues surrounding an incident are resolved. If individuals perceive that they are not acted on, they will not report adverse incidents. A common comment from health professionals is that 'nothing gets done about it'. This shows a negative feedback where poor resolution can impact reporting. Quite often incident reports are collected and stored . Rarely is benefit garneted from its

wealth of information to address underlying safety issues. A system that ensures that results from analysis are followed until closure, ensures management accountability and valuable feedback to all staff.

SUMMARY

- Clinical Risk Management encompasses a range of activities which aim to develop good quality of care and safety.

- It includes preventing potential adverse incidents, learning from adverse incidents and patient's complaints and providing staff with the support to reflect and improve their practice.

- The full benefits of clinical risk management will only be achieved if there is a comprehensive and co-ordinated system and positive support for it throughout the organisation.

References

1. Donaldson, L and Halligan A. Implementing Clinical Governance : turning vision into reality-BMJ, June 2001;332:1413-1417
2. Donaldson, L.J and Gray, J.A.M (1998), Clinical governance: a quality duty for healthcare organisations', Quality in Healthcare, vol 7 (suppl) pp537 - 44
3. Davies, H.T.O, Nutley, SM and Mannion, R, (2000), Organisational culture and quality of healthcare', Quality in Healthcare, vol 9 pp111-119
4. Goodman, N.W(1998), 'Clinical governance'. BMJ, vol 317 No 7174 pg 1725-7
5. Nicholls S, Cullen R, O'Neils, Halligan A. NHS Support Team-Clinical Governance: Its origin and its foundation. British Journal of Clinical Governance 2000; 5(3) :172-178
6. Charles Vincent ,Clinical Risk Management 2nd Ed BMJ Books 2001
7. An Organisation with a Memory, Reports of CMO 2000: http://www.doh.gov.uk/orgmemreport/
8. BMJ; 18 March 2001 'Reducing Error Improving Safety' http://bmj.com/content/vol320/issue7237/
9. RCOG 2001. Clinical Risk Management for Obstetricians & Gynaecologists-Clinical Governance Practice No2 London
10. Clinical Negligence Scheme for Trusts, 2005. Clinical Risk Management Standards .NHS Litigation Authority.
11. NPSA (2003). 'Analysing Incidents to improve Safety' RCA Toolkit. NHS.net
12. Root Cause Analysis in the Healthcare : Tools and Techniques (2000) Joint Commission on Accreditation of Healthcare Organisation
13. Gt Britain 1999. NHS Executive 'HSC1999/123: Governance in the new NHS- Risk Management and Organisational Controls.
14. Making Amends, Report of CMO 2003 http://www.doh.gov.uk/makingamends/pdf/cmo
15. NPSA 2004. Seven Steps to Patient Safety. The full reference guide. London NPSA; 2004 [www.npsa.nhs.uk/sevensteps]
16. (13) Meadows S, Baker K, Butler J. The Incident Decision Tree. Clinical Risk 2005; 11: 66-8

Chapter 9
INFORMATION GOVERNANCE

Information Governance sits alongside Clinical Governance to provide a framework which brings together all of the requirements, standards and best practice that apply to handling information about patients. The framework brings together existing and new guidance such as the Data Protection Act, the Freedom of Information Act, records management and data quality.

'NHS organisations will be held accountable, through clinical governance, for continuously improving confidentiality and security procedures........'

(HSC 1999/012, Caldicott Guardians).

Information Governance helps to ensure that all employees comply with the law and best practice when handling personal and sensitive information. Examples of such governance initiatives in the NHS are the Caldicott Report, The NHSLA Risk Management Standards and The NHS Care Records Service.

- The Caldicott Report:

    This report forms part of the NHS information governance framework, which facilitates a standard based approach to information sharing. In its report, published in December 1997, the Caldicott Committee made a number of recommendations aimed at improving the way the NHS handles and protects patient information. These recommendations received widespread support and the framework established to implement them underpins many aspects of the NHS information strategy.

The Caldicott principles aim to ensure the highest levels of confidentiality and security for patient identifiable information held in the NHS. It addresses areas of concern such as keeping patients aware of what the NHS does with their information, making sure NHS staff know about their responsibilities and good practice, ensure that individual organisations have good security measures in place so that patient information is not accessible to unauthorised users.

Caldicott principles

The following six principles underpin the protection of patient information:

1. Justify the purpose
Only share patient information with someone with a justified need to know. Every proposed use or transfer of person-identifiable information should be clearly defined and guarded.

2. Only use patient identifiable information when it is essential
The need for using non anonymised data should be justified at each stage of the specified purpose for disclosure.

3. Use only the minimum amount of information needed
The minimum amount of non anonymised data is transferred or accessed as is necessary for the specified purpose for disclosure.

4. Make sure everyone understands their responsibilities
All staff handling non anonymised data should be made fully aware of their legal obligations under the relevant legislations and responsibilities to protect confidentiality.

5. Make sure the purpose for sharing is legitimate
Use and transfer of non anonymised patient data must be lawful, responsible and reasonable.

6. Make sure the law is understood and complied with.

Each organisation should have an organisational guardian to oversee access to non anonymised patient information – a Caldicott guardian.

- NHS Care Records Service

    The NHS Care Records Service will help NHS organisations in England to store patient health care records on computers that will link information together quickly and easily. The initiative follows from patient centred care which requires information to follow the patient so that it is available wherever and whenever it is needed. It has been developed because the healthcare is more complex to organise and provide, diagnosis and treatment of conditions is increasingly specialised and can involve groups of organisations and personnel working in cooperation and paper based records cannot support the increasing demand for care and its more complex administration.

    The system will hold two categories of patient information-a detailed care record and a summary care record. A unique identification code containing the patient's National Insurance number, will be used to link their health information together and ensure that it is stored correctly. The service will be implemented in stages and hoped to be fully operational across the NHS and General Practice by 2010.

    The benefits are three-fold:

    - Patient: Access to essential information so that they can manage and take some responsibility for their health.
    - Healthcare Professional: Easier access to up to date information round the clock to enable efficient diagnosis and treatment.
    - The NHS: Improved availability of information leading to increased patient confidence.

    With this proposed changes to how patient information will be stored, it is essential that all healthcare and frontline staff are fully informed of developments and how it affects their job and hence make sure that patients are aware of the new ways their information will be handled and their options for involvement.

    To find out more about the NHS Care Records Service visit: www.connectingforhealth.nhs.uk

- NHSLA Risk Management Standards for Acute Trusts

  The standards and assessment process are designed to provide a structured framework within which to focus effective risk management activities in order to deliver quality improvements in organisational governance, patient care and the safety of patients.

  A criterion assessed under the clinical care standards is clinical record keeping as follows:

  Level 1: the organisation must have approved a document for the management of risks associated with clinical record keeping.

  Level 2: the organisation can demonstrate implementation of the approved document.

  Level 3: the organisation can demonstrate that there are systems in place to monitor the overall effectiveness of the approved document for the management of risks associated with clinical record keeping.

  The following are some of the assessed criterion at level 1:

  There is a unified health record which all specialities use;

  - Records are well designed and robust so that key information can be found readily and loss of documents and traces minimised;
  - The health record contains clear instructions regarding filing of documents;
  - There is clear evidence of clinical audit of record keeping standards for all professional groups in at least 25% of specialities..........;
  - There is a mechanism for identifying records which must not be destroyed

STORAGE OF MEDICAL RECORDS

The period for which patient records are required to be kept will vary depending on legislation or guidance issued by the Department of Health (DoH). Records may be retained longer than recommended if they are the subject of litigation or ongoing research. They should be clearly marked 'not for destruction'. Most NHS organisations however tend to microfilm the records after its period of retention. Under the DoH guidance, the following category of patient's records are retained for periods as follows:

a. Children – at least to the date of the child's 21st birthday
b. Obstetrics – 25 years
c. Adult – 8 years after last treatment
d. Oncology - 8years
e. Deceased – 8 years after death

References
1. NHSLA Risk Management Standards for Acute Trusts (April 2006) London: NHS Litigation Authority
2. Department of Health (1997) The Caldicott Committee Report on the review of patient identifiable information. London HMSO
3. Health Service Circular (HSC) 1999/012 Protecting and Using Patient Information. A manual for Caldicott Guardians
4. Health Service Circular 1999/053- For the Record : Managing records in NHS Trusts and Health Authorities.
5. Medical Protection Society (1999) Medical Records - London
6. Nursing and Midwifery Council (2002) Guidelines for Records and record Keeping. London
7. www.connectingforhealth.nhs.uk
8. www.doh.gov.uk/dpa98/index.htm (2000)

Chapter 10
COMMUNICATION

Effective and good communication is essential between all doctors and staff involved in the care of the patient to protect their safety and maintain high standards of clinical care. Communication is an essential bedrock for the provision of clinical care. Clinical Governance in the new NHS quotes as one of the four main components of CG 'effective continuity of clinical care with high quality systems for clinical record keeping and the collection of relevant information'.

In order to illustrate this pervasive subject of communication, the discussion will come under the following headings - ' Defensible documentation' 'Best Practice in Record Keeping' and 'Best Practice in Handover'.

DEFENSIBLE DOCUMENTATION

The product of medical care is the patient and the medical records. Clinical records provide an objective record of the care of the patient, and are essential in keeping other professionals caring for the patient well informed. Patient health records (electronic or paper based) include medical and nursing notes, photographs/slides, microfilm, audio or video tapes, cassettes, disks, memory chips, CD-Rom, X-ray and imaging reports, results of investigations, administrative records (personnel, complaints) referral to other persons e.g GP's, Insurance Company,

Police, DVLA.

A doctor has a professional and legal obligation to keep medical records as part of the care of his patient. The duty is to 'keep clear, accurate, legible and contemporaneous patient records which report the relevant clinical findings, the decisions made, the information given to patients and any drugs or other treatment prescribed;

- to keep colleagues well informed when sharing the care of patients; communicate effectively with colleagues within and outside the team.

(GMC :Good Medical Practice 2001(para 3, 36)

Records are valuable because of the information they contain. That information is only usable if it is correctly and legibly recorded, kept up to date and easily accessible when needed. Each of these records is only as valuable as the information it contains and that is only of value if it can be found when needed and then used effectively. Each health care professional has a key role to play in maximising benefits to patient care through effective record keeping.

Good record keeping ensures that:

- you can work with maximum efficiency without having to waste time hunting for information
- others involved in the care of the patient can see what has been done, or not done and why. This is important in providing care, clinical liability, audit, teaching, disputes or legal action and investigating complaints.
- An objective record of the patient treatment is obtainable when responding to complaints, investigations, disputes and litigation.
- Auditing of records, which is an important part of the clinical governance process is facilitated.

Best Practice in Record Keeping

A patient's health record should inform any clinician who has responsibility for the patient of all the issues which might influence the treatment proposed. It should provide a contemporaneous and complete record of the patient's treatment and related events. Currently there is no single model for documenting and communicating information that forms the patient health records. Whatever format they are presented, it should give a clear picture of the doctor's involvement in the care of the patient and stand up to audit, administrative and legal scrutiny.

Patient records should:

- **Have the patient's name and hospital number clearly written on each page**
- **Be factual, consistent and accurate.**
  - record any important and relevant information making sure that it is complete and comprehensive;
  - legible so that it can be read and reproduced when required;
  - Avoid jargons and abbreviations. Abbreviations, if used should follow common conventions;
  - be written as soon as possible after the event providing current information on the patient;
  - Any subsequent addition or later entry should be documented as a separate paragraph noting the author, time and date. Scribbling in between an earlier entry is unprofessional and raises doubt as to the motive of the author. Any amendment to the notes must not deface the earlier entry by erasure or painting over. A previous entry can be cancelled by drawing a line across the entry with 'cancelled' written on the line in addition to the name of the person effecting the cancellation with the date and time.
  - Record only opinions and facts known to the author. Perjorative remarks irrelevant and offensive comments are best avoided as patients can

    request to see the notes.

- **Be relevant and useful**
  - Document the care planned, decisions taken, information given and any discussion held.
  - Be comprehensive with fuller than normal notes when there is an

adverse incident or hint of trouble ahead.

- **Timed, dated and signed with the author's name legibly printed.**
- **Should enable another colleague to construct your consultation with the patient.**

BEST PRACTICE IN CLINICAL HANDOVER

Communicating what you do, what you have done or plan to do for the patient is essential for the continuity of care, safety and wellbeing of the patient. The handover of patient care from one team or healthcarer to another is one of the most perilous procedures in medicine. If carried out carelessly or hurriedly can be a major contributory factor to subsequent error and harm to the patient. Everyday, doctors and nurses handover information about patient care to one another. Handover is a dual process between the team handing over and the team taking over.

The changing pattern of how doctors work from the individual doctor based approach to a team based approach, on-call to full/partial shift rotas means that individual continuity of care is extinct. As a consequence of these changes, robust handover mechanism are now of the utmost importance for patient safety. Good handover practice should have a protected scheduled time, place and defined leadership. The fundamental aim of any handover is to achieve the efficient transfer of comprehensive clinical information at times of staff changes.

One of the agenda of Clinical Risk Management is to create and maintain safe systems of patient care. A fundamental strategy in this agenda is effective communication. The facilitation of high quality handover should be part of the clinical governance issue at all levels. There is clear evidence that poor quality handover is a significant risk to patients. The CESDI 7th & 8th Annual Reports highlighted two recurring themes where communication between health professionals and patients contributed to suboptimal care. The Department of Health Report 'An Organisation with a memory' cites an example involving the death of a patient consequent to poor communication amongst the medical staff. Although a number of system failures were identified, it was noted that there was no formal face to face handover between the doctors involved.

COMMUNICATION

The following is a guidance for doctors for best practice in handover. Full details of the guidance is available on 'Safe Handover': Safe patients: Guidance on Clinical Handover for Clinicians & Managers BMA 2004. http://www.bma.org.uk/ap.nsf/content/handover

I. Good handover does not happen by chance. It requires cooperation from all those involved in the care of the patient.
   - Shifts must coordinate
   - Adequate time must be allowed
   - Handover should have clear leadership
   - Adequate information technology support must be provided

II. Sufficient and relevant information should be exchanged to ensure patient safety.
   - The clinically unstable patients are known to the senior clinicians.
   - Junior members of the team are adequately briefed on concerns from previous shifts, referrals, transfers and admissions.
   - Tasks not yet completed are clearly understood by the incoming team.
   - 'Outlies' i.e. patients admitted to wards outside the teams usual wards must be notified to all members of the team.

III. A plan of team action should be formulated.
   - Tasks should be prioritised
   - Plans for further care are put into place
   - Unstable patients are reviewed.

Effective and safe handover mechanisms have the following benefits:

Patient benefit:

- Safety is protected
- Less discontinuity of care, fragmentation and inconsistency
- Decreased repetition means patients are less irritated by having to go through their medical histories over and over again.

Staff benefit:
- Educational: better handover will be of daily benefit to practice and helps the development and broadening of communication skills. A well led handover session provides a useful setting for clinical education.
- Professional protection: Clear and accountable communication can protect a doctor against blame for errors which occur.
- Reduction of stress: We can all identify with the frustration felt when the patients' records are inadequate or lacking. Having the information and feeling informed allows doctors to feel supported and on top of the patients care.

Common Pitfalls During Handover

- Verbal handover can lead to valuable information being lost. Ideally the team handing over should submit a written update and checklist to the team taking over. Otherwise the latter team should take written notes from a verbal handover. The importance of written handover must be emphasised as they provide important sources of information for the team taking over care of the patient. It also reduces the time spent searching for information.
- Roles and responsibilities are not always clear during handover and this can lead to omissions. Every team handing over must define who has the responsibility of updating the team taking over the care of the patient. The current practice of handover from SHO to SHO / SpR to SpR is less than ideal as it has a risk of fragmentation of information. Multidisciplinary team handover is preferable including the nursing staff as well. This will ensure a seamless flow of information.

SUMMARY

- Good doctor to doctor handover is vital to protect patient safety.
- Multidisciplinary handover is important to ensure all groups of staff are updated with current patient information.
- With the increase in shift pattern of work, the importance of good handover has never been so crucial.
- Systems need to be in place to enable and facilitate handover.
- Continuity of care is paramount to protect patient safety;
- Continuity of information is essential to continuity of care

SAFE HANDOVER = SAFE PATIENTS

Reference

1. For the record: Managing records in NHS Trusts and Health Authorities: HSC 1999/053: Appendix A: Dept of Health guidelines
2. Safe Handover = Safe Patients . Guidance on clinical handover for Clinicians and Managers- BMA 2004 http://www.bma.org.uk/ap.nsf/content/Handover
3. Clinical Risk Management 2nd ed, Charles Vincent BMJ Book 2001
4. An organisation with a memory; Report of CMO 2000, http://www.doh.gov.uk/orgmemreport
5. Reducing error; improving safety. http://bmj.com/content/vol 320/issues 7237/
6. Making Amends, Report of CMO 2003 http://www.doh.gov.uk/making amends/pdf
7. GMC: Good Medical Practice 3rd Ed May 2001
8. GMC: Confidentiality; Protecting and Providing Information April 2004
9. GMC: Seeking Patient Consent : The Ethical Considerations Nov 1998
10. Nursing & Midwifery Council: Guidelines for Records & Record Keeping April 2002
11. Health Professional Council : Distillation of Standards relating to record Keeping. Nov 2003
12. Department of Health HSG (96) 18 'The Protection and Use of Patient Information'

Chapter 11
PERFORMANCE MANAGEMENT

The clinical governance policy emphasises the notion that staff working in the NHS need to have the right skills for the job they do. Within the framework, professional self regulation and lifelong learning are key features. There is a duty on health professionals and teams to maintain skills, keep up to date and be aware of their skills and training needs to ensure that they have the appropriate skills and competencies. This is essential to improve quality of care and patient safety. Clinical tutors must ensure that infrastructure to ensure educational and governance activities are well supported. Organisations have a duty to ensure that knowledge and information is made available to staff with appropriate modern technology.

New training needs are constantly being identified to improve service deliver and ensure that the right learning and development is available and accessible to all staff.

Further there are training requirements to meet professional, legal and service delivery. There are five key areas namely:

a. Statutory training – There is a legal requirement to fulfil these. Examples include fire drills, Equal opportunity and race equality, disability discrimination.

b. Mandatory training – This is training that all staff are obliged to undertake as governed by the Trust for the Trust to meet other legal requirements as a corporate body. Examples include cardiopulmonary resuscitation, anaphylaxis, manual handling and lifting, child protection and protection of vulnerable adults.

c. Professional Training – this is the statutory training required by the professional body. Examples include laparoscopy training, advanced life support training, management of obstetric emergencies, neonatal resuscitation.

d. Service training – this is decided at local level in order to enable staff understand the work and system of work. These training should be in line with the skills and knowledge framework.

e. Developmental training – this is personal development training which is optional and at the discretion of the individual. Examples include MSc, MD programmes

Doctors have a professional obligation to 'keep your knowledge up to date throughout your working life. In particular, you should take part regularly in educational activities which maintain and further develop your competence and performance' (GMC: Good Medical Practice 2001, para 10-11).

CONTINUING PROFESSIONAL DEVELOPMENT

Continuing Professional Development (CPD) is underpinned by the GMC's guidance 'Good Medical Practice' (2001), which describes the principles of good medical practice, and standards of competence, care, and conduct expected of doctors in all aspects of their professional work. These include good clinical care, maintaining good medical practice, teaching and training.

There is increasing pressure on healthcare professionals to ensure that their practice is based on evidence from good quality research and stay well informed on developments in specialist areas. Clinicians need to appreciate that to provide quality care they will need to examine their own practice continually in the light of new information. This is underpinned by professional and contractual obligations.

Within the clinical governance framework, continuing professional development is a key element to support staff with the appropriate skills, training and information technology if they are to practice well. Staff development programmes must be patient centred , build on previous knowledge, skills and experience and focus on the development of clinical teams.

A record of the CPD/CME activities undertaken should be kept as well as any difficulties in attending CPD/CME activities. These records will form part of the process of an appraisal.

Managing Poor Performance

Matters of under performing medical and dental staff has become increasingly important both from a Clinical Governance perspective and the use of inappropriate suspensions in such cases. The majority of performance issues can be successfully addressed through counselling and educational remedial processes.

Managers handling matters of performance improvement need to recognise the distinction of a formative (educational) and normative (disciplinary) process and have in place appropriate systems to deal with each. The application of a disciplinary process to achieve performance improvement is detrimental and cannot achieve the desired effect.

Cases of unsatisfactory performance of doctors are dealt with under a Department of Health framework 'Maintaining High Professional standards in the modern NHS' as set out in the document Restriction of Practice and Exclusion from work Directions 2003. The Direction introduces the first two parts of a new framework for handling concerns about the conduct and performance of medical and dental staff. It covers action to be taken when concern is raised and whether there needs to be restrictions placed on their practice.

From April 2004, all NHS bodies must comply with the 'framework' and have procedures for handling serious concerns about an individual's conduct and capability. Concerns about doctors and dentists in training should be treated as training issues and the post graduate deanery involved. Where there are questions of professional competence, a disciplinary procedure is not appropriate at the outset. Trusts should explore how to improve professional competence through training opportunities. Allegations of personal conduct will continue to be dealt with using the disciplinary procedure as for all other staff. Matters of professional conduct or competence must be dealt with under the nationally agreed procedures.

The new framework recognises the continuing development of the National Clinical Assessment Service (NCAS), a division of the National Patient Safety Agency and emphasises the central role of the NCAS in helping Trusts to deal with issues of professional conduct and capability. Investigations into concerns about a doctor or dentist's practice will be handled by appropriately trained individuals locally. The advice of the NCAS should always be sought on options to resolve the matter. The formal procedure is to convene a capability hearing involving the doctor, executive and non executive directors with a clinical and human resources input. The doctor will be able to respond to any investigation report, question any witnesses and be accompanied by a companion. The outcome of any investigations should be discussed with the doctor concerned. A range of options should be explored such as no case to answer, re-education, supervision, mentoring, referral to Occupational Health Department should be explored. If there is no agreement on a plan to resolve any identified problems or on referral to the NCAS, then the Trust may have to consider disciplinary action or referral to the G.M.C.

Summary of Key Action

- Clarify what has happened and the nature of the problem concerned.
- Discuss with the NCAA what the way forward should be.
- Consider whether restriction of practice or exclusion is required. If a formal approach under the conduct and capability procedures is required, an investigator should be appointed.
- If the case can be progressed by mutual agreement, consider whether an NCAA assessment would help clarify the underlying factors that led to the concerns and assist with identifying the solution.

APPRAISAL

With the increasing emphasis on staff competencies and patient safety, appraisals have been put in place for the review of staff performance and to inform their continuous professional development. It is a fundamental component of the clinical governance strategy to help prevent doctors developing problems. For NHS doctors, appraisal will be the method for gathering revalidation evidence and a powerful indicator of a doctor's current fitness to practice. Evidence of participation in the appraisal process will show the GMC that the doctor is discussing the quality of his or her own work and keeping up to date.

Its aim is essentially developmental:

a. To identify areas of personal and professional development needs, career paths and goals;

b. To agree plans for them to be met;

c. Provide an opportunity for reflection and reassurance;

d. To optimise the use of skills and resources in achieving the delivery of high quality care;

e. To offer an opportunity for doctors to discuss and seek support for their participation in activities.

Appraisal is about feedback and reviewing an individual's performance over a defined period, with a view to identify that person's training needs, construct and agree a development plan – it is part of a doctor's career development.

The process of appraisal should embody a positive and developmental approach, be fair, effective and well informed. It should be :

i. A constructive dialogue between the appraised and the appraiser

ii. A means to discuss staff contribution to quality improvement

iii. An opportunity to discuss how the service objectives will be met and what skills need to be developed .

iv. It should leave the appraisee valued with clear objectives.

The appraisal should include data on clinical performance, training and education, audit, concerns raised and serious clinical complaints, application of clinical guidelines, relationships with patients and colleagues, teaching and research activities, and personal and organisational effectiveness. The doctor undergoing appraisal needs to prepare an appraisal folder demonstrating information, evidence and data to inform the process. Every appraisee must have a Personal Development Plan (PDP). This should identify and set out the key development objectives for the year ahead which relate to the appraisee's personal and or professional development. It will include action identified in the process of appraisal, job planning and other development activities.

To be effective and constructive to the CG agenda, it should not be bugged down with paperwork, bureaucracy or witch hunt as these will drive out the developmental aspects.

Chapter 12
COMPLAINTS

Formal complaints against doctors are now common place as to justify a knowledge of the procedure that follows the event. With increasing emphasis on accountability and ownership, every healthcare professional should be equipped with the skills and diplomacy to handle queries and complaints from patients. Whilst complaints that refer to a particular individual are taken personally, general complaints that refer to systems and dissatisfaction with the services are often 'disowned' as belonging to the management. Complaints are no longer the responsibility of the 'manager', but all staff should be involved in dealing with them effectively and learn lessons from them. All healthcare staff should understand the complaints process and the need to handle complaints effectively as part of good client care.

Complaints often arise when patients are not kept informed or involved in their car, failures in communication and lack of respect. Complaints provide important information about patients' experiences and therefore lessons can be learnt from the experience of patients who raise concerns. This concept if embraced in a non adversarial approach, the information obtained can be used to identify wider issues and trends to raise standards.

The complainant can avail themselves of any of the options of the NHS Complaints process, professional regulatory body (e.g GMC) or The HealthCare Commission to lodge their grievances. This chapter will focus entirely on the NHS and GMC complaints procedure. The scope of the issues of the complaints will relate to either conduct or performance in the clinical setting.

The NHS Complaints Procedure

The detail of the legal framework for the NHS complaints procedure is set out in the Regulations laid by the Department of Health- NHS (Complaints) Regulations

SI 2004 1768. Under these Regulations,

- Each NHS body must make arrangements for the handling and consideration of complaints (s3(1))
- The arrangements must be accessible and as such as to ensure that complaints are dealt with speedily and efficiently (s3(2))
- Each NHS body must designate a person, in these Regulations referred to as Complaints Manager, to manage the procedure for handling and considering complaints (s5(1))

Stage 1- Local Resolution

Local resolution aims to resolve complaints quickly and as close to the source of the complaint as possible using the most appropriate means. The new NHS complaints procedure places a huge emphasis on local resolution whenever possible. This procedure covers complaints made by a person about any matter connected to the provision of NHS services by the NHS organisation or primary care practitioner. The procedure also covers services provided overseas or by the private sector where the NHS has paid for them. The complaint is made in the first instance to the organisation or primary care practitioner providing the service.

The time limit for local resolution is 25 working days. If the matter is not successfully resolved at this stage the complainant has the right to have their complaint reviewed at the second stage. This must be within two months of receiving a final, formal written response from the organisation or practitioner about whom the complaint was made.

Stage 2 – Independent Review

In August 2002, The Department of Health decided that the second stage of the procedure should be removed from the local NHS body as was previously the case and give it to an independent organisation, The Healthcare Commission.

The HealthCare Commission (HCC) independently review NHS complaints at the second stage. HCC intends to establish and operate a demonstrably independent, consistent and timely process. They have a wider range of options to resolve the complaint. Mechanisms are in place to identify recurring issues or clusters of complaints against a particular individual or hospital. These will be related to other parts of the HCC surveillance mechanisms to ensure that they are put in the wider context. Anonymised reports of all HCC investigations and panel hearings are available on their website. Complaints that cannot be resolved at this stage may be referred to the next stage either by HCC or the complainant.

Stage 3 – The Health Service Ombudsman

The Ombudsman is completely independent of the NHS and the Department of Health. Its role include the investigation of clinical complaints, whether the complaints procedure itself is working or complaints where the NHS body has refused to investigate the complaint on the basis that it is outside the time limit.

The Ombudsman can also investigate complaints from NHS staff if they feel that they have suffered hardship or injustice as a result of the procedure, provided that established grievance procedures have been followed and the persons remain dissatisfied.

The GMC Complaints Procedure

From November 2004 the GMC introduced a new single complaints procedure. All complaints relating to health, performance or conduct will go through the same process. This means that a robust view is taken of the doctor's fitness to practice irrespective of the underlying cause. The same outcome and actions will be available to apply to every case as appropriate. Council members will no longer sit on the panel to decide the case against a doctor but a panellist who is appropriately assessed for suitability. This new system will streamline the current processes and ensure that complaints are processed as promptly as is consistent with achieving fairness.

When can the GMC take action?

Full details of the guidance for doctors referred to the GMC is set out in the GMC guidance - A guide for doctors referred to the GMC (Nov 2004) www.gmc-uk.org/standards. This guide explains how the GMC deals with concerns about doctors that have been referred to it by patients, employers, the police and other bodies.

The GMC will take action if the doctor's fitness to practice is impaired for any of the following reasons :

– Misconduct

– Deficient performance

– A criminal conviction or caution

– Physical or mental ill health

– A decision by a regulatory body in UK or overseas

– Significant departure from the principles set out in the Good Medical Practice

Procedure

The procedure considers the nature of the concerns and the evidence to assess what action, if any, may be required. There are 2 stages :

- 'Investigation' The complaint is assessed to see whether there is a need to investigate further ,and if so, what form the investigation should take. If the GMC decision is to investigate, the doctor will be informed of same and given an opportunity to comment on the issues. The employer will also be asked if they have any concerns in order to obtain a fuller picture of the fitness to practice. The investigation will depend on the nature of the concern raised and the investigation team will decide on the most effective form of the investigation. An investigation may include obtaining further documentary evidence from the employer, complainant and other parties, witness statements, expert reports on the matter, an assessment of the doctor's performance or health. At this stage it may be necessary to restrict or suspend the doctors registration if it is considered necessary to protect the patient, in the public or doctor's interest. If that is the case the doctor is referred to the Interim Orders Panel (IOP). The outcome of the investigation includes no further action, a warning, undertakings on health and performance issues and referral to the Fitness to Practice panel.

- Adjudication: This stage consists of a hearing of the cases which have been referred to the Fitness to Practice panel. The panel consists of specially trained people who will hear all the evidence and decide whether they need to take action regarding the doctor's registration. The panels are normally held in public except where the consideration is about a doctor's health. If a complaint is referred to the panel, the doctor will be informed in writing setting out the specific allegations and explaining the processes involved. Doctors appearing before the panel must seek legal advice and assistance from their defence organisation or specialist employment law solicitor. Where the panel make a finding that the doctors fitness to practice is impaired, it may put conditions on the doctors registration, suspend the doctor or remove the doctor from the medical register.

- Appeal: A doctor has 28 days in which to appeal to the High Court or Privy Council against any decision by the Fitness to Practice panel. During the appeal period, the panel can still impose an immediate order of suspension or conditions in the interest of the public or the doctor.

Chapter 13
MANAGING A COMPLAINT

Observational evidence suggests that many patient complaints are triggered by inadequate explanation of what happened when the patient was in hospital or failure to explain at all. There is an exponential rise in the complaints received from patients and therefore all doctors will sooner have to respond to one. Following a formal complaint or an adverse incident, a request is made to the doctor for a response or a statement. This can cause much distress or aggravation but you must remain objective and rational about it. This means trying as much as possible to understand why there is a complaint and not just what is being complained about. The process may also be part of the risk management and national patient reporting policies to identify system and human causes and drive changes in order to avoid a repetition.

The GMC provides guidance on the obligations of a doctor during a complaints and enquiries procedure in its booklet 'Good Medical Practice' (2001) paras 29-32

- Patients who complain about the care or treatment they have received have a right to expect prompt, open, constructive and honest response...para 29.

- You must cooperate fully with any formal enquiry into the treatment of a patient and with any complaints procedure which applies to your work.......para 30.

Before responding to a complaint and or writing a statement, it is helpful to discuss the content of your response with a work colleague who is not involved in the incident. Additionally guidance can be obtained from the British Medical Association, or any of the defence organisations if you are a member. The following are some practical steps to note before responding to a complaint or request for statement:

- Obtain the clinical notes and refresh your memory. This is why notes written contemporaneously with the event is helpful. Don't forget that you may be writing this statement months or years after the event when memory will have faded. If it comes to light that erroneous or misleading facts have been entered either by yourself or another party or you recall further facts then a separate entry should be made stating the date and time of the entry. No attempt should be made to add or erase anything from the original notes recorded.

- Relive the event in your mind: date, time and venue, what and what did not happen, all the parties present.

- The statement is about your involvement! The function of the statement is to relate the facts. Avoid irrelevant statements, opinions and views about what should have been done. State what you or any other parties involved in the care did. Where it is necessary to express an opinion, especially where it is difficult to separate this from a fact, it should properly relate to the clinical scenario and based firmly on what you personally perceived. Where you have no knowledge of a matter, simply state so. Avoid personal or derogatory comments about anyone as this can appear as 'mud-slinging', unprofessional and defensive.

PRIVILEGE

Privilege refers to immunity from disclosure of a document. Legal professional privilege exists to protect the right of any person to obtain advice about the law effectively and without fear that the advice may afterwards be disclosed and used to his prejudice. Documents protected by legal professional privilege fall into two categories:

a. Advice Privilege – Letters and other communications passing between a party and his solicitor are privileged from disclosure provided they are written by or to the solicitor in his professional capacity and for the purpose of obtaining legal advice or assistance for the client.

b. Litigation Privilege – Communications between the solicitor and a third party that come into existence after litigation is contemplated or commenced and they are made with a view to litigation. Examples are witness statements and expert reports.

Following an adverse incident, reports and statements compiled for the purpose of incident reporting, investigations and risk management do not attract privilege status. As the statements are often prepared even before any contemplation of litigation they are not 'privileged' materials. They are therefore subject to scrutiny by the other party in the event of litigation. It is therefore imperative to be mindful of its contents especially with incriminatory statements, personal comments and unsupported opinion.

Writing a statement 'dos' and 'don'ts'.

DO's
1. The statement should be in a chronological order of times and dates. It should have a heading stating the name and designation of the doctor, patient name and hospital number it relates to. Preferably it should be word processed, with double line spacing, signed, dated and name clearly printed.
2. Prepare a statement as soon as possible after the event.
3. Stick to the facts. Make clear what is from memory and what is from recollection of standard practice at the time.
4. Keep it simple. Do not use legal terminology e.g liability
5. Provide a chronological account of the entire course of events. Include all relevant and factual information such as the state of affairs on the day e.g workload, staffing levels. Describe actions taken by yourself and that of others witnessed by yourself. Do not report on hearsay evidence or gossip.
6. Respond within the deadline . If this causes a problem contact the

person who requested the report.

7. If responding to a complaint or inquiry, make sure you have responded to all relevant points.
8. Be honest, not defensive or evasive.
9. State your full name and qualification.
10. Sign, date and keep a record of your statement and relevant parts of the patient's notes.

DON'Ts

1. Just regurgitate what is in the case notes
2. Speculate on what others were doing or thinking unless you know something as a fact.
3. Give opinions or blame on the care given by other clinicians.
4. Attempt to write statements in a hurry or without access to all medical records.
5. Be hostile, rude or unnecessarily defensive
6. Delay in responding thinking it will 'go away'. (it will only come back in flames!)

Suggested Format for writing a Statement

STATEMENT

Name ---

Job Title ---

Date of Incident --

Time of Incident --

Location of Incident --

Statement Regarding:

Patient Name:

Hospital No:

This statement is written from extracts of …………(refer to any written records used) / recollection of events / usual course of practice.

Signed: ------------------------   Date: -------------------

Contact details (bleep no, telephone no etc)

Chapter 14
DEALING WITH AN ADVERSE INCIDENT

The increasing complexity of medical procedures means that ever than before things will go wrong despite active risk management policies. An adverse incident is anything less than is expected in the outcome of medical care. The nature of the incident whether minor or serious will depend on the nature of the outcome or complication arising. This will include a 'near-miss' where no harm has occurred to the patient but there has been a catalogue of human or system failure.

The following is action plan for guidance only, to be followed after an adverse incident:

- Call for help as soon as possible particularly if emergency treatment is needed for the patient's care. It may be prudent for the doctor involved to step aside and let others manage the situation or at least take a less active role. This is to avoid making errors of decision in an emotional/distressed state. Depending on the seriousness of the situation the most senior doctor available in the unit should take lead of the clinical scenario.

- The Consultant should be informed either immediately or in the aftermath of the incident depending on the seriousness of the situation. In a serious adverse incident the Consultant should see the patient with the utmost exigency, to offer support to the patient and input to the plan of management.

- The patient and or the next of kin must be informed of what has happened and the plan of action. A skeletal explanation may suffice at this stage as it may be necessary to conduct further investigations and later give a fuller explanation. This avoids premature or erroneous statements being made which may cast doubt on any findings made later. If conflicting explanations are given, it fuels suspicion of mismanagement, leading on to complaints and litigation. Any explanation should be made by the person most appropriate to do so and clearly recorded.

- A record of the incident must be made contemporaneously with the event. It should detail the clinical findings, any investigation or treatment given as well as the rational for these. The date and time of the event must be included as well as the name and signature of the author. If notes are written later it must be clearly stated as such with the time of writing and the time of the event . As part of record keeping and the risk management policy, an Incident Report form should be filled.

- A debriefing meeting should be held either immediately or at a later date chaired by the lead Consultant. Meeting with the doctor/s involved in the incident is helpful as a form of Root Cause Analysis technique. This is to identify the fundamental cause(s), what lessons can be learnt and associative corrective action that if rectified, will prevent recurrence of the adverse incident. This provides the insight needed to develop effective error reduction strategies and solutions.

- A meeting with the patient is an essential part of the follow up of the adverse incident. This should ideally be done as soon as possible after the event, by the Consultant or very senior member of the team explaining what has happened. In some cases a later meeting may be necessary pending the outcome of investigations and results. Whatever the information disclosed, it should be done compassionately, and sensitively. Be honest and open about what has occurred and what is being done to prevent recurrence.

- An immediate apology is not an admission of guilt or legal liability. It shows openness, will stem the anger of the patient/carers and often diffuse a prickly situation. The lack of explanation, an apology can be perceived as being arrogant and can be a powerful stimulus to complaint or litigation.

There is an ethical and professional obligation to inform the patients of adverse outcomes. 'If a patient under your care has suffered harm, through misadventure or for any other reason, you should act immediately to put matters right, if that is possible. You must explain fully and promptly to the patient what has happened and the likely long and short term effects. When appropriate you should offer an apology'. (GMC: Good Medical Practice (para 22, 23)

The National Patient Safety Agency (NPSA) has developed a 'Being Open' policy for healthcare organisations outlining how they should set in place systems to facilitate openness between staff and patients/carers following an incident.(www.npsa.nhs.uk/health/resources/beingopen).

In line with the agency's drive to help the NHS move away from asking 'who did it' to 'why did the individual act in this way' when things go wrong, the NPSA has designed an e-based interactive tool to help NHS managers dealing with staff who have been involved in a patient safety incident - The Incident Decision Tree. The aim is to promote fair and consistent staff treatment between healthcare organisations. The Incident Decision Tree complements the NPSA's Root Cause Analysis toolkit.

For both the patient and the health professional, adverse incidents can lead to much pain, anguish and uncertainty. Patients want an apology and an explanation of the incident that has occurred and what is going to happen to them afterwards. The staff involved in an adverse incident can also experience profound consequences particularly if blame is attributed rightly or wrongly. The clinician needs support and clarity as to the administrative process that follows the event. It is therefore essential that each NHS organisation should have in place support systems to deal with queries and fears and the health professional can feel encouraged to talk about their concerns. Finally each organisation should ensure consistency in the approach to dealing with communication, investigations and normative or formative process to deal with the health professional involved.

Chapter 15
DISCIPLINARY AND GRIEVANCE PROCEDURES

Disciplinary and Grievance procedures are formal routes for the employer and the employee respectively to raise and resolve disputes and concerns. The Employment Act 2002 (Dispute Resolution) Regulations 2004 SI 2004752 sets out the statutory guidance for these procedures. The essence of the Act is that employers and employees will be required to follow a minimum three stage process to ensure that disputes are discussed at work. The process requires that:

a. the problem is set out in writing with full details provided to the other party;
b. both parties meet to discuss the problem and
c. an appeal to be arranged if requested.

One underlying purpose of the proposal is to provide increased protection to employees. A failure to follow the statutory disciplinary and grievance procedure where they apply will be penalised by the Employment Tribunal.

DISIPLINARY PROCEDURE

Disciplinary Rules and Procedures help to promote civil employment relations, fairness and consistency in the treatment of individuals. It makes work rules clear and informative. The procedures should have personnel development at its centre. Employees should be informed of conduct which constitute gross misconduct and the likely consequences of a breach. It is imperative on the employer to list examples of acts of gross misconduct that may warrant summary dismissal.

A disciplinary procedure is triggered by acts of misconduct. Misconduct covers a multitude of sins of an action whether done in the course of employment or not, as to reflect in some way on the employer/employee relationship. It is unlikely that any set of rules will cover all possible disciplinary issues, but rules normally cover:

- bad behaviour such as fighting or drunkenness
- unsatisfactory work performance
- harassment or victimisation
- misuse of company facilities e.g. e-mail, telephone, internet
- poor time keeping and unauthorised absence
- breach of confidentiality
- disobedience to reasonable instruction

In dealing with matters of misconduct two approaches are used depending on whether this is a first minor misconduct or a repeat of a minor misconduct or a gross misconduct.

Informal approach: Minor misconduct are usually dealt with informally. This usually takes the form of a verbal caution. If the formal approach is not achieving the corrective outcome or the matter is more serious, then a formal approach is adopted.

Formal Approach: Conduct constituting gross misconduct are those resulting in a serious breach of contractual terms. The standard statutory procedure to be used in almost all cases is set out in full in schedule 2 of the Employment Act 2002.

It requires the employer to:

1. Inform the employee in writing of the allegations against them, the basis of the allegations and invite them to a meeting to discuss the matter.

2. Hold a meeting to discuss the allegations at which the employee has the right to be accompanied. The employee should be allowed to set out there case and answer any allegations that have been made. The employee should also be allowed to ask questions, present evidence, call witnesses and be given an opportunity to raise points about any information provided by witnesses. Following the meeting the employer must decide whether disciplinary action is justified or not and the employee should be informed.

3. If the employee wishes to appeal against the decision in (2), the employer must hold an appeal meeting at which the employee has the right to be accompanied.

The range of responses of the employer following a disciplinary meeting include:

I. Written warning- this will usually apply to cases of minor misconduct. A written warning is part of the formal disciplinary process and the consequence is a change of behaviour. Failure to change could be a final written warning and ultimately dismissal. A record of the warning is usually kept and disregarded for disciplinary procedures after a specified period e.g. 6 months

II. Final warning- failure of a change in behaviour following a written warning or an offence which is sufficiently serious may warrant a final written warning. It will give details of and grounds for the complaint and consequences of failure to improve or modify the behaviour, usually dismissal.

III. Summary dismissal- if the employer considers the conduct of the employee as gross misconduct, he may summarily dismiss. This is dismissal without notice or pay in lieu of notice.

DISCIPLINARY AND GRIEVANCE PROCEDURES

Exclusion from work

The employer may exclude the employee from work with full pay if he considers it helpful or necessary. In cases involving gross misconduct, where relationships have broken down or there are risks to an employer's property or responsibilities to other parties, exclusion from work will be appropriate whilst investigations are carried out.

When serious concerns are raised about a doctor's practice, the employer must consider whether it is necessary to place temporary restrictions on their practice. This might be to amend or restrict their clinical duties, or provide for the exclusion of the doctor. The decision to exclude can be a knee jerk reaction made by management without sufficient investigation. In certain cases it may be protective to the doctor who is emotionally distressed and unable to safely perform their clinical duties. Exclusion from work should only be imposed after careful consideration and should be reviewed regularly. It should be made clear that it is not a disciplinary action.

GRIEVANCE PROCEDURE

Grievances are concerns, problems or complaints that employees raise withy their employers. The grievance procedure is used by the employer to deal with the employee's complaints fairly, consistently and speedily so that complaints are properly considered. As much as possible, employees should aim to resolve most complaints informally with their line manager. This allows for problems to be resolved quickly and preserve interpersonal relationships. It is more expedient to raise the grievance and deal with it before the employee leaves the employment. There is a statutory procedure which the employee must adhere to in raising a grievance formally with management. A summary of this is set out below ,the full details are found in schedule 2 of the Employment Act 2002.

1. Inform the employer of the grievance in writing.

2. The employer will hold a meeting to discuss the grievance. There is a right to be accompanied to the meeting and be notified of the decision in writing.

3. An appeal process if not satisfied with the outcome of the grievance meeting.

References:

1. Maintaining High Professional Standards in the Modern NHS : A framework for the initial handling of concerns about doctors and dentists in the NHS – Dept of Health HSC 2003/012.

2. Employment Act 2002, schedule 2, paras 1-8

3. Employment Act 2002 (Dispute Resolution) Regulations 2004 (SI 2004/752)

4. ACAS code of Practice – Disciplinary & Grievance Procedure 2004 PI

APPENDIX A

SYNOPSIS OF THE ENGLISH LEGAL SYSTEM

The aim of this chapter is to give the reader a cursory understanding of the English legal system and the reporting of legal case law. This handbook can only be properly understood and be meaningful to the reader if there is an appreciation of the legal process and case reporting- unmasking the veils of mystery and tradition which shroud the English legal system. The outline described here is that which obtains in England and Wales. Scotland and Northern Ireland have a separate system.

The Sources of the Law

There are two main sources of the law- Legislation and Case law.

Legislation

The House of Parliament passes law on any subject in the form of legislation- An Act of Parliament which lay down what can and cannot be done. An Act of Parliament is sovereign over other forms of law in England & Wales i.e. can completely supersede any judicial decision or previous Act of Parliament. An Act of Parliament is referred to as primary legislation. The interpretation of these laws is the remit of the judges. Parliament may delegate the role of making the law to public bodies especially the local authority. This is known as delegated or secondary legislation. They have the same force of the law as an Act of Parliament. There are three types of delegated legislation- Orders in Council : by the Queen and the Privy Council to make laws

- Statutory Instruments : rules & regulations made by the government ministers. Statutory Instruments often contain the words Rules, Regulations or Order in their title.

- Byelaws: made by local authorities to cover matters within their remit.

Examples:

An Act of Parliament (primary legislation) e.g Human Rights Act 1998

A secondary legislation – Statutory Instrument known by the abbreviation

SI e.g. National Health Service (Venereal Diseases) Regulations 1974

The HMSO website – www.hmso.gov.uk contains the full text of SI's from the beginning of 1987 and text of Acts from 1988 onwards.

Case Law

Case law otherwise known as common law is the basis of English law today. It is unwritten law that judges have developed over many centuries through the decision in cases that have come before them where there is no governing statute.

Common law is built on the doctrine of precedent on the understanding that judges in the higher courts (Court of Appeal & House of Lords) have supremacy over the lower courts(County Court & High Court). Decisions of the House of Lords are binding on the lower courts below it and can also overrule earlier decisions on similar fact case in the Court of Appeal. The Court of Appeal decisions are binding on the lower courts if the House of Lords has not ruled on a similar case earlier. Decisions of the High court or County court are not binding on other courts or the same courts.

The Doctrine of Precedent

The English system of precedent is based on the notion 'stand by what has been decided and do not unsettle the established' This provides for fairness and certainty in the law. If a point of law in a case has never been decided before then the decision will form a new precedent for future cases to follow. In such circumstances the judge is likely to look at cases which are the closest in principle and may decide to use similar principles. This way of arriving at judgements is called reassuring by analogy.

Precedent can only operate if the legal reasons for past decisions are known. Therefore at the end of a case the judge will give a speech giving the decision and the reasons for that decision. The reasoning will explain the principles of law applied in arriving at the decision. These principles are known as the 'ratio decidendi' which means the reason for deciding. These principles create a precedent for deciding future cases. The remainder of the judgement is known as 'orbiter dicta' i.e. other things said and do not have to be followed in future cases.

A binding precedent is created in similar facts cases and the decision was made by a court which is senior to the court hearing the case.

STRUCTURE OF THE COURTS

The English legal system has a recognisable hierarchy with the senior courts hearing more important and appeals from the lower court with House of Lords being the highest court. The United Kingdom being part of the European Community, EU laws have supremacy over U.K laws including Acts of Parliament. Legal rulings must be compatible with the European Convention of Human Rights and the House of Lords is subject to the European Courts of Justice.

Some courts will only hear civil cases, others criminal cases and some will hear both.

The hierarchy in civil cases is as follows:

> European Courts of Justice (ECJ)
>
> House of Lords
>
> Court of Appeal
>
> High Court
>
> County Court
>
> Magistrates' Court

The hierarchy in criminal cases is :

> European Courts of Justice (ECJ)
>
> House of Lords
>
> Court of Appeal (Criminal Division)
>
> High Court   (Divisional Court)
>
> Crown Court
>
> Magistrates' Court

- The House of Lords

    This is the second chamber of the House of Parliament and most senior national court in the legal system. The House of Lords is the final appeal body for all civil and criminal cases though its decisions may be referred to the European Courts of Justice. The House of Lords hears appeals from the Court of Appeal and by a special procedure directly from the High Court. The House of Lords is not bound by its own decisions although it will generally follow them. It must however follow the decisions of the ECJ.

    The judges in the House of Lords are called Law Lords. There must be at least three judges for a sitting to be quorate although in practice appeals are heard by five judges up to a maximum of seven. This allows for a majority decision to be made. There may therefore be more than one judgement . In particularly important cases or a complicated point of law, more than one judge may want to explain his legal reasoning on the point.

    Cases heard in the House of Lords will be reported as:

    Bolitho v City and Hackney HA [1997] 4 ALL ER 771, HL

- The Court of Appeal

    This is the second tier of appeals in England. It has two divisions- the civil and the criminal division. It hears appeals from county courts, the civil decisions of the High Court and various tribunals e.g employment. Many more appeal cases come to the Court of Appeal than the House of Lords and so decisions here set most of the precedents that have to be followed by the lower courts and from which the common law is built. Three Lord justices make up a court and are decided by a majority of judges (2-1). The judge who disagrees will have given his reasons referred to as a dissenting judgement . If the case goes on to the House of Lords, it is possible that the House of Lords may prefer the dissenting judgement and decide the case in the same way.

    Cases heard in the Court of Appeal will be reported as:

    Airedale NHS Trust-v- Bland [1993] AC 789

Appendices

- The High Court

The Divisional Courts of The High Court

The term Divisional Court is used when one of the three divisions of the High Court (see below) acts as an appeal court.

The High Court hears the more important and expensive civil cases. The cases are usually heard by one judge. The High Court is bound by all higher courts and in turn binds lower courts. It comprises three courts as follows:

– The Queen's bench (QBD)   (Kings Bench depending on the gender of the monarch)
This is a civil court for claims worth over £15,000. There are two specialist courts within the QBD for commercial and maritime disputes. An important function of this court is Judicial Review- a review of the administrative decisions taken by public authorities. The application for judicial review is a particular procedure by which a litigant can seek review of a governmental decision. In medical matters, this would be applications by patients to obtain court declarations on the decision of a health authority to provide or not some form of medical treatment .(e.g Mrs 'S' against Swindon Health Authority to provide the cancer treatment Herceptin) (unreported Times 12th Feb 2006)
Judicial review cases are reported as:
R v A (respondent body) ex parte B (the applicant)

– Chancery Division
This deals with 'equity' matters such as mortgage repossessions, wills and administration of estates, administering the affairs and property of the mentally incapable (Court of Protection). In medical matters examples would be applications by a hospital to provide or withdraw medical treatment to incompetent adults.

– Family Division
These hear family disputes- defended divorces, custody of children, local authority care applications, maintenance and adoption matters.
In medical matters these would be applications by a hospital to provide or withdraw medical treatment in the case of minors.

- The County Court

    This is the lowest rung of the civil courts dealing with smaller cases and claims worth less than £15,000.00. They deal with cases relating to breach of contract, personal injury, landlord/tenant disputes to name a few. Cases are heard by a judge (district judge or a recorder). Appeals from the county court are heard by the Court of Appeal.

- The Crown Court

    The Crown Courts hear the more serious criminal cases not tried in the magistrates court . Some offences can only be tried in the Crown court whilst some can be tried in either court. The crown court can hear appeals by defendants from convictions in the magistrates' court.

- The Magistrates' Court

    These are the most junior courts and can hear both civil and criminal cases. In civil matters, the magistrates' courts have an extensive matrimonial and family jurisdiction.

- Other Courts

    – Tribunals
    These are specially constituted bodies for deciding disputes in a particular area of law. A tribunal. Like a court can be defined as an independent, impartial body with power to make decisions binding on the parties. All tribunals have a specialised jurisdiction. For example, industrial tribunals settle employment disputes. Tribunals often consist of three people, a legally qualified chairman and two lay members with appropriate qualifications and experience. The procedures are designed to be simple, straight forward and informal as possible hence eliminating the elaborate trappings traditionally associated with the higher courts. Although tribunals are outside the conventional courts system, they are subject to control by the courts and part of the judicial system.

Appendices

- European Court of Justice (ECJ)

This is the European Union court of law. Legal decisions from U.K courts can be referred to the ECJ where it can be overruled. Decisions made in this court are binding on all courts in England & Wales, although not on itself.

- The European Courts of Human Rights

This court deals with issues of human rights. It gives rulings on whether conduct by a public body infringes the European Convention on Human Rights.

Abbreviation	Court
HL (E)	House of Lords – England & Wales
PC	Privy Council
CA Civ	Court of Appeal – Civil Division
CA Crim	Court of Appeal – Criminal Division
QBD	Queen's Bench Division
Ch	Chancery Division
Fam	Family Division
ECJ	European Court Of Justice
SC	Supreme Court

CRIMINAL versus CIVIL LAW

Criminal Law:

This sets out the types of behaviour which are forbidden and at risk of punishment.

A criminal offence is often a breach of a prescribed law to protect a person or property. e.g Offences against the Person Act 1861, Theft Act 1968. It is an offence against the state and the state has the right to bring prosecution proceedings. The main objective of criminal prosecution is to punish the perpetrator of the crime not to compensate the victim. The accused is referred to as the defendant in legal proceedings. The standard of proof is 'beyond reasonable doubt' i.e > 90% probability of guilt.

Criminal cases are reported as follows:

R v Jordan(1956)

Civil Law:

This is concerned with the rights and duties which private individuals have in relation to each other. An individual (the claimant (previously plaintiff)) sues another (the defendant) for some harm to person or property. There are several branches of the civil law. The two principal causes of action in civil cases are the law of contract which is concerned about the rules that govern the formation of contracts and the law of torts which is primarily concerned with providing a remedy to persons who have been harmed by the conduct of others e.g. medical negligence. The aim is to obtain compensation for the person who has suffered the wrong. The standard of proof is 'on the balance of probabilities'.

Overview of the civil process

The civil courts administers redress where a civil wrong has occurred. In the civil courts the defendant will be held liable if it is shown on a balance of probabilities that he was to blame. This is lesser burden of proof than in a criminal case 'beyond all reasonable doubt'. For most purposes these two burdens of proof, it is the difference between 'definitely' and 'probably' or perhaps the difference between '90% sure' and '60% sure'.

The great majority of civil actions in the realm of medical law is clinical negligence. Negligence is injury/damage arising by the defendant doctor failing to take the sort of care a reasonable doctor would be expected to take. Negligence always requires some form of careless conduct which usually, although not necessarily, the product of inadvertence. Negligence consists of a legal duty to take care and breach of that duty by the defendant causing damage to the claimant. Proving negligence is an arduous task for the victim of a medical accident. In order for a claimant (patient) to have a successful claim in negligence the following must be proved:

a. That a duty of care exists

b. That a breach of that duty has occurred- this is concerned with the standard of care that ought to have been adopted in the circumstances

Appendices

and that the treatment fell below a minimum standard of competence

c. That he or she has suffered an injury and that the negligence must have caused the claimant's injury or that it is more likely than not that the injury would have been avoided , or less severe, with proper treatment. This limb is concerned with the causal connection between the defendant's negligence and the claimant's damage.

d. No matter how gross the defendant's negligence he will not be liable if, as a question of fact, his conduct was not a cause of the damage. It is for the claimant to prove on the balance of probabilities, that the defendant's breach of duty caused the damage.

e. The loss must be calculated in financial terms- damages.

The claimant must show on the balance of probabilities that negligent treatment caused or materially contributed to damage. Once the above have been successfully proven, compensation for damages can then be assessed. The principal remedy available to the victim of medical negligence are damages to compensate for the loss. He is entitled to be restored to the position that he would have been in, had the damage not been committed in so far as this can be done by the payment of money. The compensatory principle can be elusive in cases of medical negligence. This is due to the difficulty of placing a monetary value on physical injury and the uncertainty in predicting future prognosis, improvement or deterioration.

The time limit for making a claim is three years from the date of injury but it can be longer if:

– The patient is a child, when the three year period only begins on the 18th birthday

– The patient has a mental disorder within the meaning of the Mental Health Act 1983 so as to be incapable of managing his/her affairs, when the three year period is suspended.

– There was an interval before the patient realised or could reasonably have found out that he/she has suffered a significant injury possibly related to the treatment.

Appendix B

OVERVIEW OF A MEDICAL NEGLIGENCE CLAIM

- Pre Legal Action

  a. Requests for disclosure by the claimant or solicitors
     - Medical records to include CTG, scans, drug charts, anaesthetic records
     - Protocols and guidelines
     - Statement from staff
     - Risk Management document- Incident reports etc

  b. The claimant's solicitor sends a letter of claim to the defendant Trust
     - A letter of claim sets out the allegations, injuries and outcome
     - Likely value of the claim

  c. The defendant's solicitor sends a letter of Response within three months setting out matters agreed and matters not agreed with reasons.

- Formal Legal Proceedings

  1. Claim form and particulars of claim issued at Court. This must be accompanied with the medical reports and a schedule of loss.

  2. The defendant must file an Acknowledgement of service and Defence within the time limits for filing and respond to each allegation of negligence.

  3. The Court schedules a case management conference which sets a timetable for the procedural steps in the case e.g exchange of witness statements, Expert reports, schedule of financial losses and expenses associated with the injury costs and settlements through mediation.

  4. The Trial
     The Claimant's evidence is first
     The Defendant's evidence next
     Summing up by both sides and Judgement by trial judge.

Appendices

APPENDIX C

LEGAL CASE REPORTING

The cases reported in the law reports are commonly cases heard by the High Court, Court of Appeal or the House of Lords. This is because of their significance either the cases make new law, give a modern judicial restatement of existing principles or interpret legislation which is likely to have a wide application or clarify an important practice or procedure. Cases heard in the lower courts rarely get reported. Cases are reported in various law reports as follows:

f. The Law Reports : this includes the appeal cases, the chancery, family and Kings/Queen's bench Division (AC, Ch, Fam, KB/QB respectively) The Law Reports is the most authoritative version of a law report as it is the only series where the text of the report is checked before publication by the judges and counsel involved in the case.

g. Weekly Law Reports (WLR)

h. All England Reports (All ER)

Some law reports take precedence over others that follows the hierarchy of the courts. The above is a hierarchy of law reports.

CASE CITATION

This is the reference to find a complete report of a case. They contain the following parts:
- Year
- Volume number
- abbreviation for the law reports series
- page number on which the law report starts

Example:

1. Gillick-v- West Norfolk and Wisbech AHA [1986] AC 112

[1986] the year in which the case was reported

AC   abbreviation for the law reports series (Law Reports, Appeal Cases)

112   the page number on which the law report starts

2. Bolam-v- Friern Health Management Committee [1957] 1 WLR 582

[1957]   the year in which the case was reported

1   the volume number

WLR   Weekly Law Reports

582   the page number on which the report starts

Brackets:

[ ] square brackets mean that the year is essential to finding the case. It indicates the year the report was published.

( ) round brackets mean that the volume is more important than the year in locating the case. In these series, each volume may contain cases heard and decided in a number of different years, which is why you must rely on the volume number.

Appendices
APPENDIX D
GLOSSARY OF LEGAL TERMS

Act of Parliament: Law which is made by, or on behalf of Parliament (as opposed to case law which is made by the judges) .Also known as legislation or statute.

Binding Precedent: A previous decision which has to be followed

Breach of Duty: The standard of care that ought to have been adopted in the circumstances, and whether the defendant's conduct fell below that standard.

Civil Law: Concerns the settlement of disputes between parties which may be individuals but may include businesses and corporate organisations.

Claimant: Person who brings a claim in a civil proceeding. Previously referred to as plaintiff.

Common Law: Principles of law developed in the judgements of decided cases in contrast to statute law created by an Act of Parliament. It is also referred to as case law.

Criminal Law; Concerns the rules concerning behaviour that the state prescribes against and will punish.

Delegated legislation: Parliament has given power to a body to make specific law for specific circumstances. Also referred to as secondary legislation. E.g. statutory instruments.

Defendant: Person defending a claim.

Dissenting: A difference of opinion

Equity: Fairness

Fiduciary relationship: A position had or given in trust.

Lord Justice (LJ): Title of a judge in the Court of Appeal

Negligence: Refers to the tort whereby persons who by carelessness have caused damage to others may be held liable to pay compensation. It consists of a legal duty to take care and breach of that duty by the defendant causing damage to another.

Orbiter dicta: Used in legal judgements to refer to other thing said in the decision but do not form the principles of the decision.

Overruling: A decision which states that a legal rule in an earlier case is wrong. Only a higher court e.g. House of Lords can overrule the decision of a higher court e.g. High Court

Plaintiff: The party who brings a suit in a civil proceeding. Now referred to as claimant.

Parliament: The seat of the government. Consists of the House of Commons which has legislative functions and the House of Lords which has judiciary functions.

Reversing: Where a higher court in the same case overturns the decision of the lower court. For example the House of Lords may disagree with the judgement of the Court of Appeal and come to a different view of the law and reverse the decision of that court. Only a higher court can overrule the decision of a lower court and never vice versa.

Statute: Legislation enacted by an Act of Parliament

Tort: A civil wrong

Appendices

APPENDIX E

NATIONAL HEALTH SERVICE STRUCTURES

<u>The HealthCare Commission</u> (www.healthcarecommission.org.uk)

The Healthcare Commission (HC) is an independent body set up to promote and drive improvement in the quality of healthcare and public health. Its aims are to :

- Inspect the quality and value for money of healthcare and public health.
- Equip patients and public with the best possible information about the provision of healthcare.
- To promote improvements in healthcare and public health.

Its functions and duties are to

1. assess the management, provision and quality of NHS healthcare and public services.
2. Review the performance of each NHS Trust and award an annual performance rating
3. Regulate the independent healthcare sector through registration, annual inspection, monitoring complaints and enforcement.
4. Publish information about the state of healthcare
5. Consider complaints about NHS organisations that have not been resolved.
6. Promote the coordination of reviews and assessments carried out by the Healthcare Commission and others.
7. Carry out investigations of serious failure in the provision of healthcare.

<u>The National Patient Safety Agency</u> (NPSA) www.npsa.nhs.uk

The National Patient Safety Agency (NPSA) is a special health authority created to coordinate the efforts of the entire country to report and more importantly to learn from mistakes and problems that affect patients. The NPSA encourages all health

Care staff to report incidents without undue fear of personal reprimand. One of its key objectives is to transform the prevailing culture of blame into a culture of safety and openness. The NPSA's work now encompasses:

I.   Safety aspects of hospital design
II. Cleanliness and food
III. Ensuring research is carried out safely through its responsibility for the Central Office for Research Ethics Committee (COREC)
IV. Responsibility for the National Clinical Assessment Service (NCAS) (formerly the NCAA) which addresses concerns about the performance of doctors and dentists.

The NPSA helps the NHS learn from things that go wrong and develops solutions to prevent harm in the future. It works with patient and staff locally and nationally to foster a culture where errors can be investigated and innovative solutions developed. It collects and analyses the information from staff and patients via the National Reporting and Learning System (NRLS) and other sources.

The NLRS is one of the major achievements of the NPSA to date. The system is designed to draw together reports of patient safety errors and system failures from health professionals across England and Wales to help the NHS learn from things that go wrong.

National Clinical Assessment Service (NCAS)   www.ncas.npsa.nhs.uk

The National Clinical Assessment service is a division of the NPSA, set up as one of the central elements of the NHS modernisation plan to ensure the high quality of healthcare. NCAS was previously the NCAA , a special health authority until April 2005 when it became part of the NPSA.. NCAS is an advisory body that provides advice , takes referrals and carries out targeted assessment where necessary to help doctors and dentists in difficulty. NCAS also helps NHS organisations improve local management of performance concerns so that difficulties are recognised and addressed before they become more serious problems.

Central Office For Research Ethics Committee (COREC)
www.corec.org.uk

The Central Office for Research Ethics Committee working on behalf of the Department of Health in England :

1. Coordinates the development of operational systems for Local and Multicentre Research Ethics Committee (LREC's and MREC's) in the NHS;

2. Maintains an overview of the operation of the research ethics system in England, and alerts the Department of Health and other relevant authorities if the need arises for them to review policy and operational guidance relating to Research Ethics Committee and manage Multicentre Research Ethics Committee in England.

National Institute for Health and Clinical Excellence (NICE)
www.nice.org.uk

In April 2005, the National Institute of Clinical Excellence joined with the Health Development Agency to become The National Institute for Health and Clinical Excellence (also to be known as NICE to create a single excellence in practice organisation). NICE is an independent organisation for providing national guidance on the promotion of good health and the prevention and treatment of ill health. Currently NICE provides guidance in three areas of Health namely:

I. Technology appraisals- guidance on the use of new and existing medicines and treatments within the NHS in England and Wales;

II. Clinical guidelines – guidance on the appropriate treatment and care of people with specific diseases and conditions within the NHS in England and Wales;

III. Interventional procedures – guidance on whether interventional procedures use for diagnosis or treatment are safe enough and work well enough for routine use in England, Wales and Scotland.

National Health Service Litigation Authority (NHSLA) www.nhsla.com

The National Health Service Litigation Authority (NHSLA) is a special health authority responsible for handling clinical negligence claims made against NHS organisations in England. A key function of the NHSLA is to contribute to the incentives for reducing the number of negligent or preventable incidents. This is achieved through an active risk management programme to help raise standards of care in the NHS and hence reduce the number of incidents leading to claims.

The Clinical Negligence Scheme for Trusts (CNST) provides an indemnity to members and their employees in respect of clinical negligence claims arising from events which occurred on or after the 1st of April 1995. It is funded by contributions paid by member Trusts and is often equated to an in-house mutual insurer.

The NHSLA handles negligence claims against NHS bodies through five schemes- three of these relate to clinical negligence claims and two relate to non-clinical risks such as liability for injury to staff and visitors and property damage. When a claim is made against a member of the Trust, the NHS organisation remains the legal defendant. NHSLA takes over full responsibility for handling the claim and meeting the associated costs.

The risk management programme is provided by a range of NHSLA standards and assessments known as CNST Standards and Assessments. This is the core of the risk management programme of the NHSLA. Member NHS organisations are regularly assessed against a series of risk management standards which have been specifically developed to reflect issues which arise in the negligence claims against NHS bodies.

There are five sets of standards reflecting the different organisational, clinical and non clinical risks faced by different kinds of healthcare organisations:

- NHSLA General Clinical Risk Management Standards

    This standards of performance assessment falls into five categories as follows:

    1. Governance

    This standard ensures that :
    – there is an organisation wide risk management strategy

Appendices

- there is an audit committee and board sub-committee with responsibility for risk.
- the organisation has an approved document for the systematic identification, assessment and analysis of all risks (clinical, operational and corporate)
- the organisation has a risk register
- there is risk management awareness and training for all board members and senior manager
- the organisation has approved a document for the management of risks associated with records both clinical and non clinical.

2. Competent and Capable staff

This standard assesses that there are management systems in place to ensure the competence and appropriate training of all clinical staff. It ensures that there are:

- appropriate employment checks
- up to date professional registration of medical staff
- induction for temporary and permanent staff
- risk management training for all staff
- training in infection control, moving and handling

3. Safe Environment

- This standard assesses that there are processes in place to manage risks associated with:
  personal safety of staff, patients and property
- protection of vulnerable adults and children
- management of risks associated with moving and handling
- slips, trips and falls involving staff and patients
- sharps injury
- maintenance and decontamination of reusable and other medical devices
- bullying and harassment at work
- work related stress

- staff on long term sick leave

4. Clinical Care

This standard assesses to ensure that there are processes for the management of risks associated with :

- patient identification
- informed consent
- patient information on the scope of their treatment
- clinical record keeping
- reporting of clinical investigations e.g. x-rays, CT
- medicines
- blood product, handling and administration
- resuscitation procedures
- infection prevention and control
- discharge and transfer of patient

5. Learning from experience

This standard focuses on how Trusts ensure that lessons are learnt and patient care is improved through the effective reporting of adverse incidents and near misses in healthcare. It ensures that :

- there are procedures to report incidents
- service users have suitable information of procedures to register formal complaints and feedback on the quality of services
- all reported incident, complaints and claims are investigated
- there is a systematic approach to encourage learning from incidents, complaints and claims
- there are processes to ensure that alerts , notices and other communications are implemented within the required timescale.

Appendices

- agreed best practice and guidance is taken into account
- staff involved in traumatic or stressful incidents, complaints or claims are adequately supported
- all communication is open, honest and occurs as soon as possible after the event.

- CNST Maternity Standards
  This assesses the way risk management activities are organised in these important services, focussing on areas such as communication, clinical care, and staffing levels.

- CNST Mental Health and Disability Learning

- NHSLA Standards for Primary Care Trusts
  This applies to all PCTs. It assesses such factors as incident reporting and investigation, infection control, health records and the validation and monitoring of professional registrations.

- NHSLA Ambulance Standards
  This aims to ensure that each Ambulance Trust as part of its system of internal control embed a rigorous Risk Management process that covers all risks.

Clinical Governance Support Team   www.cgsupport.nhs.uk

This is a multidisciplinary team set up to support the implementation of Clinical Governance (CG) in the NHS. It offers practical support through its development programmes, information about Clinical Governance, lessons from development work across the country and a place to find answers to Clinical Governance questions.

APPENDIX F

DUTIES OF A DOCTOR REGISTERED WITH THE G.M.C

Patients must be able to trust doctors with their lives and wellbeing. To justify that trust, we as a profession have a duty to maintain a good standard of practice and care and to show respect for human life. In particular as a doctor you must:

- Make the care of your patient your first concern;
- Treat every patient politely and considerately;
- Respect patients' dignity and privacy;
- Listen to patients and respect their views;
- Give patients information in a way they can understand;
- Respect the rights of patients to be fully involved in decisions about their care
- Keep your professional knowledge and skills up to date;
- Recognise the limits of your professional competence;
- Be honest and trustworthy;
- Respect and protect confidential information;
- Make sure that your personal beliefs do not prejudice your patients' care;
- Act quickly to protect patients from risk if you have good reason to believe that you or a colleague may not be fit to practice;
- Avoid abusing your position as a doctor;
- Work with colleagues in the ways that best serve patients' interests.

In all these matters you must never discriminate unfairly against your patients or colleagues. And you must always be prepared to justify your actions to them.

Appendices

APPENDIX G
THE GMC GUIDANCE LIBRARY

The GMC publish and regularly review guidance for doctors on standards of professional conduct. The following is a list of the guidance currently available at www.gmc-uk.org/guidance/library.

Core guidance

Good Medical Practice (May 2001)
The Duties of a doctor (1995)
Confidentiality: Protecting and Providing Information (April 2004)
Research (Feb 2002)
Seeking patients' consent: the ethical considerations (Nov 1998)
Serious Communicable Diseases (1997)
Withholding and withdrawing life-prolonging treatments: Good practice in decision-making (2002)
Management for Doctors (2005)

Supplementary Guidance

Accountability in Multi-Disciplinary and Multi-Agency Mental Health Teams (2005)
Antenatal Testing for HIV (2000)
Doctors shouldn't treat themselves or their families (1998)
Giving expert advice (1998)
Guidance for doctors who are asked to circumcise male children (1997)
Intimate examinations (2001)
Good practice in prescribing medicines (2006)
Making and using audio and visual recordings of patients (2002)
Media inquiries about patients (1996)
Referring patients with personal injuries (2002)

APPENDIX H

GUIDANCE FOR HEALTH PROFESSIONALS ON COMPLETING THE DEPARTMENT OF HEALTH/ WELSH OFFICE CONSENT FORM 1

This guidance is provided for health professionals obtaining patients' consent for procedures. It follows the structure of the Department of Health consent form. Its aim is to ensure that all patients are given consistent and adequate information. You should explain the following whilst completing the corresponding section of the form.

Name of proposed procedure or course of treatment

Name and briefly explain the intervention and state the reasons it is being offered (i.e for the treatment of [name of condition or disease]).

The proposed procedure

You should describe to the patient what the procedure is likely to involve, including:

- Expected length of stay in hospital
- Medication
- Anaesthesia
- Surgery (including site and size of any incision and any likely scarring);
- Pain
- Recovery
- Likely impact on daily and personal life (e.g time off work, lifting, exercise)
- Tissue or organ removal
- Tissue examination (storage/disposal)
- Video or photographic recording

This information should be supported by dedicated patient information.

Appendices

Intended benefits

Clearly describe to the patient how she can expect the intervention to help the condition or illness.

Serious or frequently occurring risks

In order to ensure that patients understand the level of risk involved, it is best to avoid using verbal descriptions (e.g. high/low risk) or expressions of percentages when discussing risk. It is preferable to use natural frequencies and express risk in relative terms (e.g. if 100 people have this procedure, five of them will have this complication) You should bear in mind that individuals (both clinicians and patients) vary in their perception of and attitudes to risk.

You should also inform the patient of any risks associated with her own health and medical history, record them on the form, for example, obesity, previous surgery, pre-existing medical conditions, smoking, etc. The patient should be given the opportunity to discuss her own additional risks with another appropriate medical specialists if so wishes before consenting.

If a clinical department or an individual surgeon has robust data for their own complication rate, this should be given alongside national figures. It is recommended that clinicians make every effort to separate serious from frequently occurring risks.

Serious risks

Serious risks, which occur with varying frequency in certain circumstances in a pelvic operative procedures are:
- Death
- Venous thrombosis/pulmonary embolism
- Return to theatre
- Trauma to bowel, bladder and ureter.

Reference should also be made to risks specific to the planned procedure

Frequent risks

Frequently occurring risks include:
- Infection
- Bruising
- Scarring
- Adhesions
- Bleeding
- Anaemia as a result of haemorrhage

Any consequences specific to the intended procedure should be described.

Any extra procedures which may become necessary during the procedure

Blood transfusion

Inform the patient of the frequency of blood transfusion being required during or following specific operations and record this on the consent form.

Other procedures

Explain to the patient that, during a procedure, complications may sometimes arise whereby, if no further procedure is performed, the patient's life or quality of life could be compromised.

What the procedure is likely to involve, the benefits and risks of any available alternative treatments, including no treatment.

You should already have:
- Described to the patient what the procedure is likely to involve
- Provided the patient with information on alternative interventions (such as other medical, surgical or less invasive procedures) and their benefits and risks
- Discussed with the patient the risks and benefits of having no treatment.

These points should be reinforced at the time of signing of the consent form.

Appendices

Information leaflet

You should provide the patient with relevant supporting information about the procedure (either in writing or in another format appropriate to the patient's needs) and record this on the consent form.

Anaesthesia

You should inform the patient of the type of anaesthesia to be used and that she will have an opportunity to discuss it in more detail with an anaesthetist before the procedure.

Statement of patient: procedures which should not be carried out without further discussion

Ensure that the patient tells you of any specific procedures which she does not wish to be carried out without further discussion and that these are recorded.

APPENDIX I

CHILD PROTECTION

Healthcare professionals with substantial contact with children should appraise themselves with the relevant child protection training within their Trusts. This is essential in order to develop a greater knowledge of the signs and symptoms of abuse, knowledge in the identification and referral of children at risk of significant harm, ensuring diversity and ensuring that all children are treated equally.

PRINCIPLES WHICH UNDERPIN CHILD PROTECTION POLICIES

- The welfare of the child is the paramount consideration at all times
- Children should be safe and protected by effective intervention if they are in danger
- Agencies should work in partnership with parents in so far as it does not prejudice the welfare of the child.
- Children should be kept informed about what happens to them and their wishes and feelings taken into account (considered in the light of their age and understanding). They should have the opportunity to participate in decisions made about their future.
- Parents continue to have parental responsibility in relation to their children, even if their children are no longer living with them. They should be kept informed about their children and participate in decisions made about their future.
- Parents with children in need should be helped to bring up their children themselves.

ACTION TO BE TAKEN TO PROTECT CHILDREN

Step 1	Practitioner has concerns about child's welfare
Step 2	Practitioner discusses with Manager
Step 3	Still has concerns

Appendices

Step	Practitioner refers to Social Services, Following up in writing within 48hrs
Step 5	Social Worker and Manager acknowledge receipt of referral and decide on next course of action
Step 6	Feedback to referrer
Step 7	Initial assessment required
Step 8	Concerns about child's immediate safety

APPENDIX J
POST DEATH INVESTIGATIONS

The Office of the Coroner
The office of the coroner is an extremely old one . Its modern day relevance of the coroner is to inquire into the cause of certain types of death. It is an inquisitorial process and the coroner is concerned only with how the death occurred and does not seek to establish liability or causation. The investigations in the form of an inquest offer an important opportunity to gain evidence on the cause of death. The inquest is perceived by interested parties, usually relatives of the deceased, as a facilitative forum for establishing the truth. The coroner is responsible for the inquest procedure and is an independent judicial officer. The coroner must be professionally qualified for five years as a solicitor, barrister or a doctor.

When does the coroner become involved
The coroner is required to hold an inquest into deaths where there is a reasonable cause to suspect that the death is:
a. violent or unnatural
b. sudden and of unknown cause;
c. in prison or elsewhere in circumstances where another Act of Parliament requires an inquest to be held.

The construction of natural or unnatural death has been the subject of judicial contentions. In the context of medical practice, this will include deaths due to anaesthesia, accidents in hospital, poisoning, want of attention at birth, suicide, any death that has been caused by any medical or surgical treatment, or its complications

Even if the treatment was given more than 24hours before death. acute and chronic drug abuse to name a few. Commonly the coroner will decide that a post mortem should be held to help determine if an inquest should be held.

Appendices

Death Certificates

Every death has to be registered within 5 days with the Registrar of Births, Marriages and Deaths. Any doctor who has attended the deceased during his last illness must fill out a death certificate which states to the best of his knowledge and belief the cause of death. The doctor (usually now the bereavement officer) must also give the person who has to register the death (usually a relative) a written notice of the certificate, which identifies the cause of death as detailed on the certificate.

In cases that fall within the coroner's jurisdiction, this should be reported to the coroner's officer and hence the death cannot be registered until the coroner has completed his investigations. The certification of the death by a medical practitioner does not restrict the jurisdiction of the coroner as the Registrar may refer the matter to the coroner.

ORDER FORM
I/We wish to request [   ] copy(ies) of The Medico-Legal Handbook for Doctors
At £9.99 plus £1.50 (postage & packaging) per copy.

I enclose a cheque for [   ] made payable to 'thelegaldoc'.

Name ....

Address ....

....

....Postcode ....

Tel No...

Email address ....
If you are interested in medico-legal training for your organisation please use this form to request further information.

Please return this form to: The Administrator, Thelegaldoc, P.O.Box 570
Waltham Cross, Herts, EN8 1AE or email info@thelegaldoc.co.uk.

- -- - *Tear off* -

ORDER FORM
I/We wish to request [   ] copy(ies) of The Medico-Legal Handbook for Doctors
At £9.99 plus £1.50 (postage & packaging) per copy.

I enclose a cheque for [   ] made payable to 'thelegaldoc'.

Name ....

Address ....

....

....Postcode ....

Tel No...

Email address ....
If you are interested in medico-legal training for your organisation please use this form to request further information.

Please return this form to: The Administrator, Thelegaldoc, P.O.Box 570
Waltham Cross, Herts, EN8 1AE or email info@thelegaldoc.co.uk.